Angiogenesis-Based Dermatology

Jack L. Arbiser

Editor

Angiogenesis-Based Dermatology

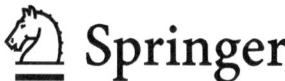 Springer

Editor
Jack L. Arbiser
Emory University School of Medicine
Atlanta, GA
USA

ISBN 978-1-4471-7312-0   ISBN 978-1-4471-7314-4   (eBook)
DOI 10.1007/978-1-4471-7314-4

Library of Congress Control Number: 2017933481

Printed on acid-free paper

This Springer imprint is published by Springer Nature
The registered company is Springer-Verlag London Ltd.
The registered company address is: 236 Gray's Inn Road, London WC1X 8HB, United Kingdom

Preface

This book is dedicated to the memory of Judah Folkman, MD, with whom I had the pleasure of spending a 4-year postdoctoral fellowship, between the years 1994 and 1998. There are several aspects to Dr. Folkman's personality that made him so effective in advancing angiogenesis in medicine. First, his research was clinically driven. He wanted to use angiogenesis as a tool to cure human disease. Thus, he chose to use basic research to address clinical problems, not as an end to itself. There are two camps of people who perform basic research with regard to human disease. The first believes that we have to know everything in order to treat human disease. A corollary of that belief is that once we know everything, we will be able to design a specific targeted therapy that cures advanced cancer or other ailment, with no side effects. This will be accomplished because advanced cancers are addicted to an oncogene, and targeting that oncogene will lead to a painless cure. The second camp is the one that Dr. Folkman belonged to, in that he wanted to know how we could leverage the knowledge that we have today to help patients who are sick today. As a pediatric surgeon, he recognized that patients who are sick today need treatments today, and will likely not survive until that utopian time that we have magic bullets with no side effects. His concepts of angiogenesis inhibition, first expounded in *The New England Journal of Medicine* in 1971, were fiercely attacked both at home and in other institutions. He had the courage to take these to clinical trials, which were also controversial, but led to new treatments of cancer and disorders of excess vasculature. He was always in a hurry because he knew that time was short and that people are sick and don't have infinite lifespans. He was also very open minded and allowed anyone to pursue their interests as long as they were related to angiogenesis. In this vein, he provided critical advice to a generation of scientists in terms of career advancement. Finally, he was a total gentleman, and never disparaged those who attacked and ridiculed him, although we knew very well the identities of these individuals. The term "noble metal" refers to metals that are resistant to corrosion, like gold. Dr. Folkman was resistant to the corrosive environment that he lived in his entire professional life. This makes him noble.

Lab meetings in the Folkman lab were Friday mornings. I personally felt as if we were knights at the Round Table of Angiogenesis, each of us representing a separate field of angiogenesis. Studies from those heady times led to the development of thalidomide for myeloma, anti-VEGF therapy for macular degeneration, understanding of the relationship of oncogenic signaling, understanding of the biology of hemangiomas and vascular malformations, isolation of endogenous angiogenesis inhibitors, urinary detection of angiogenic biomarkers, angiogenesis and metabolism, and many other advances that are in the clinic today. Dr. Folkman had a way of quieting skeptics. When someone said, that won't work, he gave him a pen and piece of paper and told him to write it down and commit to it. I never saw anyone actually committing their skepticism to paper.

Many of us alumni in the Folkman lab wonder how he would view the world today. As someone who knew him from 1994 to the time of his untimely death in 2008 in the Denver airport, I can venture some predictions. He would be thrilled with the clinical discovery that propranolol, a very old drug, is highly effective against hemangiomas of infancy, and has been applied to this condition, even though the mechanism of propranolol against infantile hemangiomas is not fully understood. He would also be thrilled by the use of rapamycin against vascular malformations. Part of the rationale for using rapamycin on vascular malformations was our discovery that mTOR is activated in vascular malformations, which we demonstrated on paraffin samples which I had acquired while in his laboratory.

Dr. Folkman would not be surprised by the failure of the oncogene addiction hypothesis, because as a surgeon, he had seen numerous advanced tumors and intuitively knew that large solid tumors were not reliant on a single oncogene. Evidence of this are the numerous mutations and mechanisms that have been reported in Braf inhibitor resistance in advanced melanoma. He would be pleased with the use of Avastin as a treatment for macular degeneration and cancer, although he would recognize that our use of Avastin causes compensatory events in solid tumors that require further therapies, such as those that target NADPH oxidases and HIF2a, a response to chronic hypoxia. He would likely be disappointed in the failures of angiostatin and endostatin in the clinic, and would call for further studies to understand why these drugs didn't show the same effect in humans as they did in mice. He would be gratified about the role of angiogenesis inhibition in promoting antitumor immunity, and would call for combinations of angiogenesis inhibitors and checkpoint inhibitors against solid tumors. Finally, he would approve of the concept of angioprevention, the use of angiogenesis inhibitors to prevent the formation of cancer, which is widely practiced today by the public with natural products.

Every dermatologist who prescribes a drug has a little bit of Dr. Folkman in them. When we prescribe a drug, we do not know the full mechanism of the action of the drug. Doxycycline kills bacteria but also inhibits matrix metalloproteinases. Which is more important for treatment of acne and rosacea? We don't know, but we don't let our lack of knowledge serve as an excuse not to treat patients. It is my hope that the well-written chapters in this book will serve to clarify to the practicing dermatologist a more full understanding of their every day actions. Once the dermatologist in the trenches has a better understanding of what they do, they too can contribute to the immediate advancement of knowledge through keen clinical observations which can be rapidly disseminated and aid treatment of patients today.

Atlanta Veterans Administration Medical Center   Jack L. Arbiser
Atlanta, GA, USA

Contents

Contributors

Jack L. Arbiser Emory School of Medicine and Atlanta Veterans Administration Medical Center, Department of Dermatology, Atlanta, GA, USA

Ana Carolina Belini Bazan-Arruda Dermatology, Hospital e Maternidade Celso Pierro – PUC-Campinas, Campinas, Brazil

Yihai Cao Department of Cardiovascular Sciences, University of Leicester and NIHR Leicester Cardiovascular Biomedical Research Unit, Glenfield Hospital, Leicester, UK

Department of Microbiology, Tumor and Cell Biology, Karolinska Institute, Stockholm, Sweden

Julide Tok Celebi Department of Dermatology, Department of Pathology, Icahn School of Medicine at Mount Sinai, New York, NY, USA

Lawrence S. Chan Department of Dermatology, University of Illinois College of Medicine, Chicago, IL, USA

Department of Microbiology/Immunology, University of Illinois College of Medicine, Chicago, IL, USA

Medicine Services, Jesse Brown VA Medical Center, Chicago, IL, USA

Captain James Lovell Federal Health Care Center, North Chicago, IL, USA

Carol Cheng Brigham and Women's Hospital, Harvard Institute of Medicine, Department of Dermatology, Boston, MA, USA

Justin Elsey Emory University Hospital, Department of Dermatology, Atlanta, GA, USA

Shoshana Greenberger Sheba Medical Center, Department of Dermatology and Sheba Cancer Research Center, Ramat-Gan, Israel

Omer Ibrahim Cleveland Clinic Foundation, Department of Dermatology, Cleveland, OH, USA

Sherrif F. Ibrahim Assistant Professor, Department of Dermatology, Division of Dermatologic Surgery, Wilmot Cancer Center, University of Rochester, Rochester, NY, USA

Lasse Jensen Department of Medical and Health Sciences, Linköping University, Campus US, Linköping, Sweden

Department of Microbiology, Tumor and Cell Biology, Karolinska Institute, Stockholm, Sweden

Wangcun Jia Beckman Laser Institute, University of California, Irvine, Department of Surgery, Irvine, CA, USA

Larissa Mondadori Mercadante Dermatology Resident, Hospital e Maternidade Celso Pierro – PUC-Campinas, Campinas, Brazil

Jiaqi Mi Medical College of Georgia, Augusta, GA, USA

Martin C. Mihm Brigham and Women's Hospital, Harvard Medical School, Department of Dermatology, Boston, MA, USA

J. Stuart Nelson Beckman Laser Institute and Medical Clinic, University of California, Irvine, Departments of Surgery and Biomedical Engineering, Irvine, CA, USA

Rebecca A. Pankove Emory University School of Medicine, Department of Dermatology, Atlanta, GA, USA

Shikha Rao Emory School of Medicine, Department of Dermatology, Atlanta, GA, USA

Vivian Y. Shi Department of Dermatology, University of Illinois College of Medicine, Chicago, IL, USA

Daniela Melo Siqueira Dermatology Resident, Hospital e Maternidade Celso Pierro – PUC-Campinas, Campinas, Brazil

Wenbin Tan Beckman Laser Institute, University of California, Irvine, Department of Surgery, Irvine, CA, USA

Huayi Zhang Department of Dermatology, University of Illinois College of Medicine, Chicago, IL, USA

Angiogenesis: General Concepts

L. Jensen and Y. Cao

Introduction

The process of blood vessel growth, generally referred to as "angiogenesis", is pivotal for the development, homeostasis and function of all tissues and organs in the organism, but also for progression of most serious diseases including ophthalmic disorders, cancer, cardiovascular disorders, inflammatory disorders and chronic skin ulcers [1]. In the last decades, great progress has been made in our understanding of the mechanisms that regulate angiogenesis and vascular functions in health and disease, and this continues to be one of the largest areas of research today [2]. It is now clear that the regulation of tissue/organ development, physiology and disease progression by blood vessels is highly complex and context-dependent, but certain general concepts and factors are central and important for angiogenesis during development and in most diseases. Such general concepts will be the focus of this chapter.

The concept of blood vessel formation and growth was first mentioned by the Greek philosopher Aristotle in the fourth century BC [3], but the concept of angiogenesis was not thoroughly studied until in the work of John Hunter who has been credited (perhaps erroneously) with introducing the term "angiogenesis" in 1787 [4]. The process and mechanisms regulating angiogenesis was however first

L.Jensen (✉)
Department of Medical and Health Sciences, Linköping University,
Campus US, Ingång 68, Pl. 08, SE-58185 Linköping, Sweden

Department of Microbiology, Tumor and Cell Biology, Karolinska Institute,
SE-17177 Stockholm, Sweden
e-mail: lasse.jensen@liu.se

Y. Cao
Department of Cardiovascular Sciences, University of Leicester and NIHR Leicester
Cardiovascular Biomedical Research Unit, Glenfield Hospital, Leicester LE3 9QP, UK

Department of Microbiology, Tumor and Cell Biology, Karolinska Institute,
SE-17177 Stockholm, Sweden

© Springer-Verlag London Ltd. 2017
J.L. Arbiser (ed.), *Angiogenesis-Based Dermatology*,
DOI 10.1007/978-1-4471-7314-4_1

systematically studied using modern in vitro and in vivo assays in the work of angiogenesis pioneer Judah Folkman [5]. Physiological, or healthy angiogenesis is mostly considered as a part of organ development, blood vessels in adults are considered to be mostly quiescent and primarily serve structural purposes as the cells forming the innermost layer of blood vessels. In pathological conditions, such as in cancer, blood vessel growth may, however, be induced in adults, a finding reported as early as in the fourth century BC by Hippocrates [5] and expanded radically in the work performed in the Folkman Lab [2]. The identification of key angiogenic factors including vascular endothelial growth factor (VEGF) in 1989 [6, 7] and the VEGF receptor (VEGFR) in 1990–92 [8–11] and their regulation, as well as the development of a palette of in vitro and in vivo assays suitable for studying mechanisms regulating angiogenesis [5] led to a more mainstream interest in the field, followed by an explosion in the number of publications related to angiogenesis in various aspects of health and disease. It is now clear that angiogenesis is important for all types of tissue growth including during development but also during regeneration of wounds or damaged myocardial or brain tissues following ischemic insults [12, 13] as well as adipose, muscle or tumor growth [14–16]. Most of the work on elucidating the importance of angiogenesis in health or disease, come from studies where the process has been inhibited and subsequent phenotypes analyzed. For example, mice lacking even just a single allele of the important angiogenic factor VEGF-A die in the womb just a few days after the first blood vessels should have been formed, due to massive vascular insufficiency, improper formation of the few vessels that do develop leading to extensive hemorrhage [17]. As a consequence of these vascular defects, mouse embryos stop developing from day E8.5, when the embryo start to require oxygen transport by its own vasculature to maintain oxygenation of the growing and developing organism, and eventually die at E10.5 [17]. Also during post-natal development VEGF-A is important for physiological growth and morphogenesis of the retinal vessels in mice [18], a process that is dependent on hypoxia-induced VEGF-A in the peripheral retina as in animals such as zebrafish that develop in the absence of tissue hypoxia, the closely related homologue VEGF-B is required for retinal angiogenesis [19]. Since these early discoveries, genetic knock-out studies have been used to identify a host of factors necessary for normal developmental angiogenesis or healthy vascular morphogenesis [20]. In addition, the potential of factors to induce ectopic angiogenesis in the otherwise avascular cornea has generated very important knowledge on factors that could be exploited for pro-angiogenic treatment [21–23] alternatively to identify the complex mechanisms involved in angiogenesis under pathological situations such as in tumors [24, 25]. In cancer, quantitative analyses of gene-expression profiles or protein abundance have identified numerous putative angiogenic factors over-expressed in solid tumors of all origins [2]. In particular VEGF-A and dual pro-angiogenic and inflammatory cytokines such as TNF-alpha [26], TGF-beta [27], various interleukins [28–30], chemokines and bone-marrow growth factors [31] as well as extracellular matrix modulating enzymes [32] have been studied along with the putative intracellular mediators. The importance of these factors have then been demonstrated by loss- or gain-of-function studies using mouse tumor models, in which tumor cells or whole animals have been genetically modified to produced pathologically relevant levels of these various factors. With so many potentially important pro-angiogenic factors identified to date, a key issue is to understand the interplay and synergistic mechanisms that drive tumor angiogenesis in complex environments where several factors are over-expressed at the same time. As such there are likely synergies between various angiogenic factors, that stem from their actions on the different cell-types needed for angiogenesis including endothelial cells, peri-vascular cells and macrophages which complicate using single specific neutralizing or agonistic agents in anti- or pro-angiogenic therapy. In keeping with this idea, single-agent treatments have largely failed both for anti-cancer therapy and for restorative angiogenesis in ischemic disorders. Combinations of pro- or anti-angiogenic drugs thus have much stronger potential in pre-clinical settings [33], but such combination therapies remains to be thoroughly tested in clinical studies.

In many cases angiogenic factors may act in a tissue-dependent manner. I.e. the factors that is important for growth of blood vessels in the brain or eye, such as Wnt7a/b, Grp124 [34, 35] or VEGF-B and Neuropilin1 [19] seem to have little if any role in angiogenesis in other parts of the organism. Similarly, factors regulating angiogenesis in the adipose or muscle tissue coinciding with the growth of these tissues in adults, may also be different from those regulating angiogenesis in for example the skin during wound healing. Leptin, produced at high amounts by mature adipocytes, is a potent angiogenic factor [36], but also more general pro-angiogenic molecules such as VEGF-A is important for adult adipose angiogenesis and blocking these factors pharmacologically inhibit diet-induced or leptin-deficiency-induced obesity in mice [37, 38].

In this chapter we aim to give an overview of the key features of blood vessels, their structure and function and how blood vessels are involved in regulation of tissue functions. In the second part we will focus particularly on the mechanisms regulating vessel growth, maturation and regression, and discuss key differences between the growth and function of healthy versus pathological vessels. Finally we will introduce the concept of lymphangiogenesis and how lymph vessels develop, function and may contribute to disease under pathological conditions.

Blood Vessel Physiology and Function

The first and foremost function of blood vessels is to supply oxygen and nutrients (mainly glucose and lipids) to support cellular metabolism. A large fraction of the blood is therefore dedicated to transport of oxygen via hemoglobin-containing erythrocytes that are responsible for approximately 50% of the blood volume. In the cell-free fraction, the most abundant proteins including albumin and lipoproteins are dedicated to transport of water in-soluble lipids/amphiphiles, and the plasma has a high buffer capacity as a way to combat acidosis or reactive oxygen species that are unavoidable side-effects from oxidative cellular metabolism. The abundance of these oxygen- or lipid-binding factors in the blood also reflect the facts that free oxygen is among the most reactive compounds in the organism and because free lipid is detrimental to vascular physiology. Blood is delivered through the

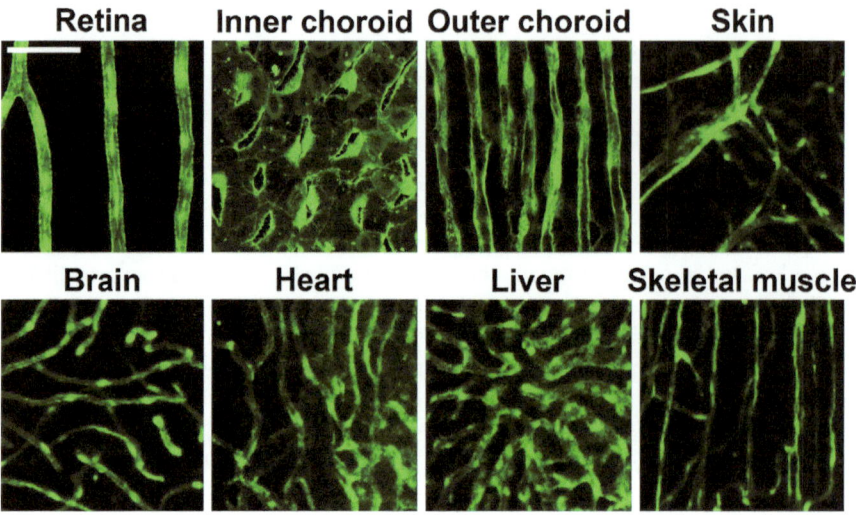

Fig. 1.1 Morphological differences between capillary beds of various tissues. Confocal micrographs of blood vessels, shown in *green*, found in the retina, inner and outer choroid, skin, brain, heart, liver and skeletal muscle of adult transgenic Tg(fli:EGFP)[y1] zebrafish, expressing enhanced green fluorescent protein (EGFP) in endothelial cells. The white size bar indicate 100 μm

vasculature to all metabolically active tissues and collected by veins which bring waste products, primarily carbon dioxide (CO_2), urea and other metabolites through the kidneys and the liver to the lungs, where the last of the waste products (CO_2) is released and the blood is reoxygenated. This constant circulation of blood is necessary for its function – blood that accumulate in tissues due to insufficient venous drainage, persistent circulation in futile loops or hemorrhage rapidly loose the tissue-supportive function and rather become a reservoir for tissue-damaging factors including cytotoxic cells and compounds [39]. As such, blood is only beneficial to tissues if it is also effectively collected and recycled.

The metabolic activity of a tissue is the primary regulator of blood perfusion. When metabolic activity increase this will lead to tissue hypoxia, which is the most important physiological signal for increasing perfusion. This is perhaps most clearly exemplified in the brain where the activity of different brain regions is directly coupled to changes in perfusion; all techniques used to measure brain activity today actually measure blood perfusion and not the activity of the nerves or other brain cells themselves [40]. In tissues which exhibit constantly high metabolic activity including the liver and the retina, blood vessel density is high compared to other tissues (Fig. 1.1). However, in tissues with dynamic metabolic activity such as the brain or muscle, the vascular density may not be particularly high but perfusion is instead regulated by changes in the vascular diameter and blood flow rates, a process known as hyperemia that can be achieved in seconds after the increased metabolic demand [41–43] – much faster and more efficient than regulating the vascular density by growth or regression of new blood vessels. As such changes in perfusion of a tissue are mainly regulated by vascular dilation/

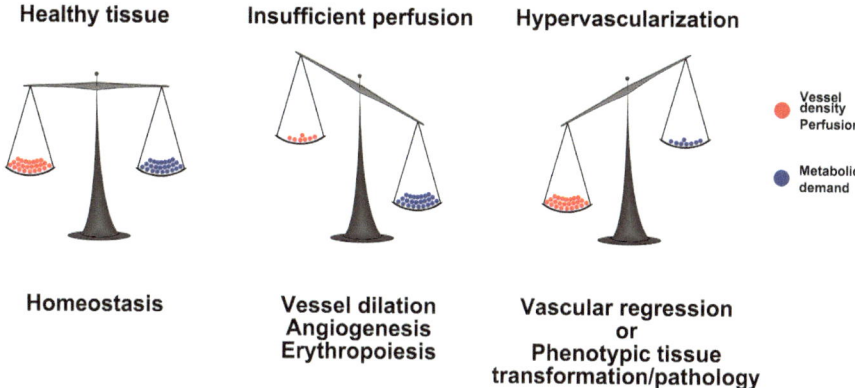

Fig. 1.2 Vascular endowment is balanced by the metabolic needs of the tissue. In healthy tissue the vessel density and perfusion (*red balls*) is balanced according to the metabolic activity of the tissue (*blue balls*; *left image*). Should the metabolism increase (*middle image*), perfusion and oxygen delivery will also increase through vessel dilation, angiogenesis and erythropoiesis. Is however the vascular density or perfusion higher than the needs of the tissue (*right image*), excessive vessels will regress or the metabolic needs of the tissue will increase (phenotypic switch). In diseased tissues, excessive vessels do not regress but rather sustain pathological transformation or growth of the tissue

contraction and hypoxia is the main physiologic mediator of these responses. On the other hand the function of a tissue also changes in response to changes in blood perfusion. For example, forced expansion of the vasculature in adipose tissue by genetic modifications leading to increased expression or local delivery of growth factors by the adipocytes, leads to a phenotypic change in the tissue from energy-storing white to energy consuming brown-like adipose tissue, with a concurrent increase in the metabolic activity of the adipocytes themselves [38, 44–46]. As such, the metabolic activity of a tissue has to be balanced by the blood perfusion, and changes in either the metabolic activity or perfusion parameter drive matching changes in the other, or lead to disease (Fig. 1.2).

Blood vessels, however, are not only a conduit for transport of oxygen, nutrients and metabolic waste products. Many factors important for organizing the functions of various organs to act in concert with each other (i.e. endocrine regulators) also use the vasculature as a route of communication and the vessels play an active role in the signaling process. For example, insulin-dependent and in-dependent glucose uptake by cells in the brain, where there is no passive leakage of glucose across the capillary, is mediated by active transport of glucose across the wall of the blood vessels by Glut1 and Glut4 glucose transporters [47, 48]. Furthermore, hormone receptors are expressed at high levels in the vessels which, in response to hormone stimulation, produce cytokines that mediate some of these hormone-dependent effects on the tissue, thus playing very important roles in endocrine regulation [49, 50]. Also under pathological conditions such as tissue inflammation, the tissue recruit immune cells to fight the inflammatory stimulus (often invaded bacteria) by activating the vessels locally, an activation that lead to the presentation of molecules including ICAM and VCAM, on the inner surface of the vessel which are recognized by the immune cells and mediate their movement across the vessel and into the tissue specifically at the site of inflammation [49]. These functions are also important for the physiologic trafficking of immune cells to various lymphoid tissues in the organism [51].

The vasculature not only transports chemicals and cells, it is also critical for the thermoregulation by transporting heat [52]. Brown adipose tissue or skeletal muscles are the main sources of heat generation due to their high expression of uncoupling proteins and inherent storage of energy either as fat or glycogen. From here, warm blood is pumped for example through the skin, which is a main tissue responsible for heat/cold sensing [53]. The important role of the blood for maintaining temperature is mirrored in the fact that core body temperature decreases during the inactive period (i.e. night in humans), when the heat generating muscle and brown adipose tissues are less active [54], although many of the other tissues exhibit similar metabolic activity.

Locally, in the tissues, blood vessels also provide key signals for the surrounding cells which are crucial for the specific function. Especially un-differentiated stem- and progenitor cells are known to exist predominantly in so-called vascular nieches, in which these cells make direct contact to endothelial cells, contacts that are crucial for maintaining the undifferentiated state of the cells [55, 56]. As such in tissues as different as the intestine, bone marrow, skin, brain and in tumors, the non-differentiated stem/progenitor cells are specifically found associated with the vasculature [57]. Also other, differentiated cells types require contact with vascular endothelial cells in order to maintain their phenotype. An example of this has recently been demonstrated in adipose tissue, where pericytes loose their identity and transform into adipocytes when their contacts with endothelial cells are disrupted [58]. Similarly, vessels-associated macrophages are primarily of the alternatively differentiated type, whereas non-vessel associated macrophages to a higher extent exhibit the classically activated phenotype [59] indicating that vessel contact may induce or maintain processes required for alternative differentiation and associated functions of macrophages.

During development, the vasculature provide key signals required for organogenesis, regulation of organ size and shape as well as differentiation and specification of cell types in the various organs. The development of the alveoli in the lungs, for example, depends on signals provided by the developing lung vasculature [60]. Should blood vessel growth be inhibited during lung development, this will lead to a failure in the development of alveoli. Also in the kidney, the vasculature provide crucial signals required for differentiation and formation of the glomeruli [61] and in the liver endothelial cells may be important for both the early development of the fetal liver, the structural development of the liver lobules and for the growth and size of the liver both during development and during regeneration [62]. Such regulatory roles of blood vessels also dominate in the regeneration of other organs and tissues, including the skin, in adults [63]. Fin regeneration in fish, for example, is stunted if blood vessel growth is inhibited leading to incomplete regeneration and a smaller fin compared to the size prior to amputation [64]. It is likely that blood vessels do more than simply provide oxygen and nutrients to the developing tissue and as such regulate its size. In zebrafish embryos, oxygenation is not dependent on perfusion during early development as the small size of the embryos allows for passive diffusion of oxygen through the tissues as the main mechanism of oxygen delivery [19]. Yet, the development of for example the kidney and liver still requires blood vessels [65, 66] indicating that there may be some still poorly characterized signals being produced by the vessels which are important for organ development.

In order to accomplish all the functions and respond appropriately to systemic or tissue-specific regulatory signals, blood vessels combine several different cell types tasked with specific regulatory properties that work together in one functional unit. Blood vessels are subdivided in three general classifications based on the direction of blood flow, pressure, vessel structure and blood oxygenation level; arteries carry high-pressure, highly oxygenated blood in an efferent manner to the tissues, capillaries are small caliber vessels that distribute the blood within and actively communicate with the tissues as described above, and veins are large caliber vessels that drain the blood from the tissues and transport it in an afferent manner back to the heart. Arteries, capillaries and veins are anatomically highly different and are also regulated differently. Anatomically, the wall of large arteries and veins may be subclassified in at least three different regulatory domains known as the intima, media and adventitia (Fig. 1.3). The innermost intima consists of endothelial cells, perivascular cells known collectively as pericytes and their shared basement membrane constructed from collagenIV, laminin, nidogen, and perlecan/proteoglycans [67]. The media (or tunica media) is a smooth muscle cell layer that covers the intima and particularly for large arteries can be many cell-layers thick and constitute the largest proportion of the vessel. Veins have thin media as the diameter of veins is to a larger extent regulated passively by the amount of drained blood rather than actively via smooth muscle contraction/dilation. The adventitia consisting of fibroblasts, connective tissue, nerves and for the largest vessels even its own vasculature (vasa vasorum) constitutes the external barrier of the vessel and is therefore the toughest part of the wall. In large arteries such as the aorta it is elastic due to the presence of elastin, which is required for the buffering of the large changes in blood pressure as the blood is pumped out of the heart. Capillaries contain only a primitive intima and generally have no media or adventitia (Fig. 1.3). Arteries and veins of different organs are rather similar in structure, function and regulation. Capillaries, however, communicate with the tissue in which they reside and are as such highly diverse depending on the needs of the tissue. For example, capillaries in the liver, glomeruli and endocrine organs such as the adrenal gland, pancreas and thyroid are very leaky due to the existence of small holes (fenesters) in the endothelium allowing small compounds and sometimes even cells to pass freely between the tissue and the vasculature [68]. In the skeletal and cardiac muscle, the capillaries are straight, and with little branching, which allow for very efficient perfusion and in the brain the capillary wall is covered with numerous other cell types including pericytes, astrocyte end-feet and even nerve endings, a structure known as the neurovascular unit or the blood-brain barrier. Also the expression profiles of the endothelial cells are different depending on the tissue, reflecting these differences in structure and function. As such, the endothelial cells of the capillaries are unique in each tissue, mirroring the specific functions of the tissue and the associated requirements for communicating with the rest of the organism via the circulation. Recently it was discovered that

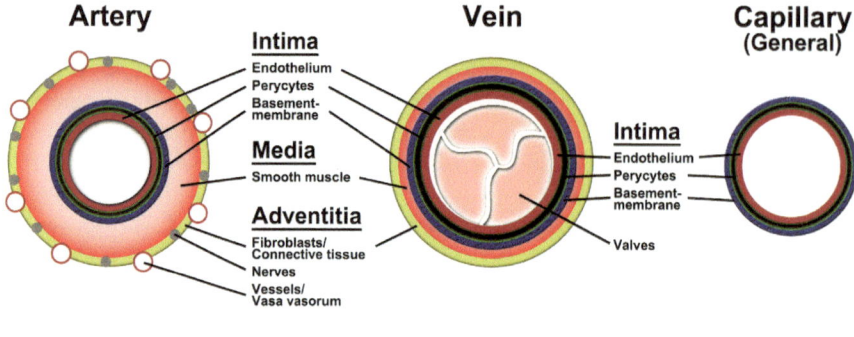

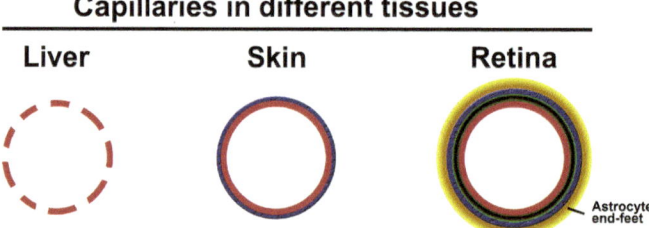

Fig. 1.3 Vascular anatomy. The anatomy of the vessel wall in large arteries, veins and capillaries are illustrated in the *top row*. The vessel wall consists of the intima (endothelial cells, pericytes and basement membrane), media (smooth muscle cells) and adventitia (fibroblasts, nerves and capillaries). Arteries have a thicker media and more nerves and vessels in the adventitia compared to veins. Capillaries lack media and adventitia. Capillaries in different tissues exhibit widely different morphologies as illustrated in the *lower row*. Capillaries in the liver (and other endocrine organs) are fenetrated and leaky, whereas a subset of capillaries in the skin lack pericyte coverage and capillaries in the brain and retina exhibit very tight and complex regulation at the vessel wall including coverage with astrocyte end-feet, giving rise to the blood-brain barrier

also the pericytes are not a homogeneous population of cells but rather that various different types of pericytes are present in the vessels and that the composition is different between organs [69, 70]. In addition, other cells such as stem/progenitor cells, immune cells and possibly other cell types may also constitute part of the wall of capillaries or larger vessels. The role of pericytes and other peri-vascular (also known as mural) cell types are poorly understood beyond that they are important for vessel stabilization and survival, but are likely important for tissue homeostasis as well as involved in pathophysiological conditions such as fibrosis, regeneration and inflammation. Possibly, some of these functions may arise from their crosstalk with endothelial cells [71], endowing the highly diversified anatomy and functions found in the capillary beds throughout the organism and as such they may be key players in tissue-specific regulation of the vasculature.

Hypoxia is the key signal for increasing perfusion to tissues. Hypoxia act via in principle three different routes; the immediate reaction is the activation of endothelial nitric oxide synthase (eNOS) activity, leading to production of nitric oxide (NO) which is one of the most potent signals for relaxing smooth muscle cells and thus dilation of arteries, via activation guanulyl cyclase-mediated cGMP production and down-stream signaling in smooth muscle cells, providing an increased amount of oxygenated arterial blood to flow into the hypoxic tissue [72, 73]. Hypoxia also lead to the increased production of erythrocytes via up-regulation of EPO in the kidneys, as well as blood vessel growth via production of vascular endothelial growth factor locally in tissues (more on this in section "Modes of Blood Vessel Formation and Regression"). This regulation is exploited pharmacologically as patients with high blood pressure are often prescribed nitroglycerin, a potent NO-donor, which will lead to vascular dilation and reduced blood pressure. In addition to direct regulation by hypoxia, blood vessels and in particular arteries are highly innervated and thus regulated by the sympathetic nervous system. As such, perfusion of muscles is enhanced under stressful situations as a part of the fight or flight response, the intestines exhibit increased perfusion shortly after meal intake, and the skin is perfused to a higher degree during exercise or in very warm or cold environments. These responses are in large part due to beta-adrenergic signaling in the neuro-vascular synapses [74]. A third important regulator of vascular function is inflammatory signaling, as sites of inflammation are hyperperfused and leaky, which is important for appropriately mounting the inflammatory defense system. In such instances, cyclooxygenase- or lipoxygenase-mediated production of prostaglandins, leucotrienes or thromboxanes, which have strong vasoactive effects, play a major role in the inflammatory vascular responses [75]. Certain neuropeptides including neuropeptide Y, vasoactive intestinal peptide, melanocyte stimulating hormone and calcitonin gene-related peptide are also important modulators of vascular function, in particular in allergies or asthma [76], in the physiologic regulation of intestinal or central nervous system perfusion. Most of these molecules act on arteries, but will lead to increased blood flow through capillaries which will activate shear-stress sensitive signaling in both down-stream arteries, pre-capillary arterioles and capillary endothelial cells. Such signaling will first and foremost lead to remodeling of the vasculature including circumferential vascular growth, vascular survival (non-perfused vessels regress over time in healthy tissues), leakage and recruitment of peri-vascular cells [77]. Shear-stress signaling however, may also lead to vascular expansion by other mechanisms, including angiogenesis, should the stimulation be sufficient to reach the pro-angiogenic threshold [78, 79], as a mechanism of providing more capillaries to absorb the increased inflow of blood into the tissue and as such reduce the pressure in the individual capillaries. The mechanisms involved in angiogenic expansion of the vasculature are the topic of the next section.

Modes of Blood Vessel Formation and Regression

Blood vessel formation can in principle be divided in two main categories – formation of new vessels by aggregation and vascular morphogenesis of endothelial cells, a process known as vasculogenesis, and the expansion of existing vasculatures, a process known as angiogenesis.

Prior to vasculogenesis, endothelial cells are specified from the hemangioblast progenitor population in the lateral plate mesoderm and migrate during early somitogenesis medially to form a main central endothelial chord [80, 81]. This process is stimulated by sonic hedgehog-mediated vascular endothelial growth factor (VEGF)-A production by the cells in the myotome and thus occurs in a central-to-rostro/caudal fashion. At this point, the endothelial cells are progenitors lacing luminal and basolateral polarization, but as they assemble and form the first vascular chord, they start to accumulate water-filled vesicles in a highly coordinated fashion in which such vesicles in neighboring cells line up with each other in a common plane. These vesicles fuse, both within each cell as well as between adjacent endothelial cells, forming the lumen of the first vessel, the dorsal aorta [82]. An alternative mechanism involving electrostatic repulsion between endothelial cells at the luminal side as a chord-hollowing mechanism has also been described [83]. Once a lumen has been formed, endothelial cells polarize and establish different functionality at the luminal versus the basolateral side, similar to the polarization of epithelial cells. The early vasculature is the site of initial hematopoiesis, where erythrocytes bud off the endothelium and are deposited as the first circulating cells in the blood islands of the yolk sac and the lumen of the aorta [84]. Concurrently, the ventral cells of the aorta also start migrating ventrally, a process that is independent of VEGF-A but instead mediated by repulsive signals between EphrinB2 expressed in the aorta and EphB4 expressed in the migrating cells [85]. These cells eventually coalesce and organize themselves with their luminal side facing inward into a large caliber vessel; the cardinal vein. These two vessels, the dorsal aorta and the cardinal vein connect to the heart and fuse to form a loop at the posterior pole at late somitogenesis stages, thus completing the primitive circulatory loop [81]. Similar processes occurs in the brain where endothelial cells arise in other mesodermal progenitor pools, migrate and coalesce to form the first cerebral arteries and veins [86]. The primitive vasculature expands by sprouting angiogenesis. The first dorsal, arterial sprouts arise at the dorsal aspect of the dorsal aorta and grow as intersegmental arteries, dorsally between the somites in a VEGF-A dependent manner [19], around the same time where the cardinal vein cells migrate ventrally. This is the first example of sprouting angiogenesis in the organism, but vascular expansion of other tissues later in development occurs by largely identical mechanisms. As such, sprouting angiogenesis is responsible for forming the vast majority of all vessels in the organism.

Sprouting angiogenesis can in principle be divided in several individual processes. As the process begins from an already perfused, and often mature, vessel, the first step is to destabilize the vessel wall by local breakdown of the basolateral basement membrane. This is achieved by induction of matrix metalloproteinases (MMPs) including MMP2 and MMP9, as well as other extra-cellular matrix (ECM) proteases [87]. In the case of vessels highly covered by pericytes, these then detach from the endothelial cells, allowing the formation of basolateral pseudopodia in the responding endothelial cells. This is followed by the induction of a tip-cell, i.e. the primary responding endothelial cell which on one hand develops large pseudopodia (filopodia and lammelipodia) allowing the cells to migrate into the tissue and on the other hand suppress similar activation of neighboring endothelial cells through the Dll4-Notch1/4 axis [88–90]. The tip cell then migrates into the tissue, scanning the path with highly dynamic filopodia as it moves and remain intimately connected to its neighboring cells which form the subsequent stalk cells. Stalk cells proliferate and as such extend the connection with the mother vessels as the tip cell drags the new vessel sprout longer into the tissue [18]. Recently, this over-simplified scheme however was revised as it was found that tip and stalk cells compete for the tip cell formation as stalk cells may move to the tip cell position and vice versa during sprout elongation [91]. As such, stalk cells may move relative to each other, but only the tip cell decide the direction of growth for the entire new vessel. When the tip cell meets with another endothelial cell, they fuse and as such terminate the growth of the vessel. This process is called anastomosis and is critical for establishing perfusion [92]. It has been suggested that this anastomosis process is regulated by macrophages which attract tip cells and mediate their fusion [93]. Following anastomosis, the two endothelial cells meeting each other form new tight junctions, which mature, remodel and modify the shape and relative position of the endothelial cells in the previously growing vessels such that their lumens are merged and blood can move between the vessels [92]. The new vessels mature by recruiting pericytes and constructing a new basement membrane which provide stability and survival signals to the vessel. These processes are however not serially induced, vessels mature as they grow and only the distal piece of the sprout is immature. Tip cells constantly secrete platelet-derived growth factor (PDGF)-B, a potent chemoattractant and growth factor for pericytes, which secure the pericyte investment of the vessel as it grows [94]. Pericytes and the endothelial cells themselves also secrete all the factors found in the basement membrane. Angiogenesis is kept in check not only by the initial restriction of sprouting by activated Notch-signaling but also during sprout/vessel elongation as the stalk cells secrete soluble VEGF receptor (VEGFR)-1, which act as a molecular trap on the sides of the vessel such that all the growth stimulatory signals are received only by the tip cells in the very front [95].

High frequency actin turn-over is important for the tip-cell function as they need to rapidly send out and retract filametous-actin rich filopodia while at the same time moving the cell forward through lammelipodia [96]. As such, small rho-GTPases including RhoA, Cdc42 and Rac which mediate the polymerization of actin, cofilin and GTPase-activating proteins (GAPs) which mediate the depolymerization of actin and Arp2/3, wasp and focal-adhesion components which mediate the structural arrangement of the actin cytoskeleton and its connection with the extracellular matrix are all critical elements necessary for sprouting angiogenesis [96]. The filopodia of the tip cells are rich in so-called patterning molecules, receptors for membrane bound ligands presented by the cells in the surrounding tissue that in the most cases exert repulsive signals on the filopodium leading to its regression. These patterning molecules in this way make sure that the vessel is not growing into tissues where it should not, but stay on its intended course [97]. This is particularly clear during development as the intersegmental vessels have a highly stereotypical shape mediated by the inter-somitic boundaries, and never grow into the somites themselves. However, in the case of animals in which semaphoring ligands or plexin receptors have been rendered non-functional genetically, vessels readily grow into the somites and the vascular development is chaotic and ineffective leading to the early embryonic demise of the animal [98]. Interestingly these patterning factors are shared by the axonal growth cones and also important for nerve pathfinding during development [97].

In the stalk cells, restraining sprouting, maintaining cell-cell junctions and proliferation are key for the extension of the vessel and maintaining its connection to the patent vasculature. Many of these aspects are regulated by shear stress as the stalk cells are carrying blood (although perfusion is poor until after anastomosis) and are thus flow-stimulated [99]. The stalk cells also express or respond to "patterning factors" such as notch and jagged but these are instead crucial for mediating the crosstalk between endothelial cells and pericytes necessary for vascular maturation. Other important factors mediating the crosstalk between endothelial cells and pericytes include angiopoietin 1 and 2, and their ligands Tie1/2 as well as transforming growth factor (TGF)beta and the TGFb receptors [100].

In addition to sprouting angiogenesis blood vessels may also grow by splitting themselves in two, a process known as intussusception. Intussusception is characterized by the local luminal bulging of the endothelium proceeding until bulges from the two opposing sides reach each other, forming a trans-vascular hole or "intussusceptive pillar", which in turn is stabilized by perivascular cells, mainly fibroblasts, moving into and filling the pillar [101]. It has been suggested that this process is primarily induced by VEGF-signaling [102], but may also be mediated by reduced notch-signaling in the endothelium, as it is the case for sprouting angiogenesis [103]. Intussusception, however, involves stalk cells rather than tip cells and the "sprouts" forming the intussusceptive pillar form on the luminal, rather than the basolateral side of the endothelium. As intussusception often lead to the formation of a loop that support circulation, this is considered a way for the endothelium to survive by enabling pro-survival shear-stress signaling under conditions of inhibited survival or growth factor signaling such as pharmacological inhibition of VEGF [104]. Some tissues, such as the lungs and the choroid in the back of the eye, however, have adopted this mode of angiogenic expansion during development [105, 106] indicating that it is also important in physiology. The intracellular processes taking place in the endothelial cells during intussusception is however poorly understood at present.

A variation of intussusception is the recently described pulling of vessels into a non- or de-vascularized area from the surrounding vascularized tissue mediated by myofibroblasts, a process that often precedes sprouting angiogenesis and is, like intussusception, dependent on myofibroblast activity [107]. This is for example seen during inflammation-induced corneal neovascularization or wound healing in the skin, where immediate vascularization of the inflamed cornea or regenerating skin is accomplished by in this way recruiting already existing vessels rather than waiting for new ones to grow [107]. It is however not known if this process plays a role during physiological neovascularization during development.

Large blood vessels are highly stable, but capillaries are constantly remodeling especially in dynamic tissues such as muscle, adipose or liver. Also during development and in wound healing/regeneration the vasculature develops as an overly dense network which then remodels to achieve its final density reflected by the needs of the tissue [108, 109]. As such, hyperoxia or hypoperfusion in blood vessels start a process of vascular regression which can largely be considered as reverse sprouting – the cell-cell junctions between two endothelial cells remodel, the lumen collapses and the junctions are dissolved leading to two tip cells being pulled backward toward the used and stabilizing vessels to which the regressing vessels connect [110]. Alternatively, in pathological situations such as in cancer or neovascular eye diseases, immature pathological vessels may also regress simply by removal of the pro-angiogenic signal, also leaving a few but much more mature vessels that are stabilized and remain in the absence of growth factor signaling [104, 111]. This ordered regression is required for avoiding hemorrhage or leakage of blood or plasma into the tissue. During regression, however, the receding vessels leave the basement membrane behind as empty sleeves, or tunnels in the tissue. Such acellular "ghost" vessels which do not carry blood, but can still be seen by immunostaining for basement membrane markers such as collagenIV, or by other types of imaging techniques, are thought to be a highway for extremely rapid neo-angiogenesis should the vessel growth signal emerge again for example during breaks in the anti-angiogenesis treatment procedure or due to recurrence of an inflammatory signal [112]. It is currently not known how this last part of the vessel, the basement membrane, is removed during developmental vascular remodeling or whether such processes could be exploited to generate more complete and long-lasting anti-angiogenic treatments in the future.

Differences in Healthy and Pathological Angiogenesis

The above description primarily pertains, in principle, to both developmental angiogenesis, constructive angiogenesis as a part of tissue regeneration as well as pathological, non-constructive angiogenesis. In pathological conditions, however, the process is deregulated in various ways, leading to formation of chaotic vasculatures that are poorly functional, i.e. tissue perfusion is often not improved, or even decreased, despite increased vascular density [113]. This leads to persistent hypoxia and further hypoxia-induced pathological angiogenesis, thus constituting a vicious circle which aggravates pathological phenotypes [114]. As such in diseases characterized by pathological angiogenesis including chronic inflammatory disorders, cancer or hypoxia-associated retinopathies such as age-related macular degeneration, diabetic retinopathy and retinopathy of prematurity, correcting the vascular function by reducing the pro-angiogenic signaling in the microenvironment for example by using VEGF-targeting drugs are in many cases effective treatments which increase the healthy functions of the inflamed or hypoxic tissue and inhibit disease progression.

A key phenotype of pathological vessels is the chaotic structure which arises from the lack of patterning signals. Many patterning factors are primarily expressed during development and are thus lacking in quiescent adult tissues [115]. While growing endothelial tip-cells re-express vascular patterning receptors, pathological tissues do not express the ligands, or the ligands are proteolytically cleaved to fragments of opposite function compared to the native molecule [116] and thus physiological vascular repulsion does not occur and vessels grow in any direction and do not follow defined trails. Another class of patterning receptor-ligand pairs, namely the semaphoring-plexin system is also involved in pathological angiogenesis, but the regulation is complicated by the fact that these protein families are rather large and different receptor-ligand interactions may exhibit opposing functions on the vasculature [117]. Nevertheless, de-regulation of the expression of patterning factors is an important, yet understudied mechanism for driving the pathological phenotypes of vessels found in inflamed and/or malignant tissues.

Under pathologic conditions, the production and secretion of angiogenic factors occurs in a deregulated manner which contributes to the disorganized overgrowth of vessels. As angiogenic stimuli are often sensed from all directions, the vessels are dragged everywhere at the same time. This is in stark contrast to the spatiotemporal production of for example pro-angiogenic VEGF in the myotome at 24 h post fertilization in zebrafish embryos, which exactly coincide with the sprouting and growth of intersegmental arteries dorsally, towards the myotomes and the subsequent repression of VEGF-A in myotome, when the vessels arrive at this location [19]. The VEGF-production is then rather shifted to the dorsal roof of the intersegmental vascular bed, leading to continued dorsal growth and eventually the formation of the dorsal anastomosing longitudinal vessel (Fig. 1.4). In pathological situations such as in cancer, the pro-angiogenic signals are not turned off or repositioned in a regulated manner, leading to vessels growing into the tissue producing the angiogenic factors and there, grow in all directions, anastomose prematurely, and immediately re-initiate sprouting in a continuous cycle leading to the formation of a vasculature characterized by highly ineffective circulation.

Persistent angiogenic stimulation also leads to defective pruning/regression of surplus or under-used vessels, a key feature of healthy vascular remodeling. Indeed, the vasculature of pathological tissues can sometimes resemble that of healthy or regenerated tissue prior to the onset of vascular remodeling in terms of containing vessels that are either non-perfused or contribute to inefficient perfusion through futile loops. High levels of proteases which are common to tissues exhibiting pathological angiogenesis prevent vascular maturation by inhibiting the formation of a continuous basement membrane and an appropriate recruitment of perivascular mural cells. The vessel wall is therefore of poor structural integrity and as a result the vessels are highly leaky and prone to disintegration leading to edema, hemorrhaging and high interstitial fluid pressure (Fig. 1.5). Such conditions further accelerate pro-angiogenic inflammation and inhibit effective perfusion leading to hypoxia [114]. Forcing vascular maturation, while leading to a stabilized vasculature that is difficult to get rid of, and which support perfusion and thereby oxygen and nutrient delivery, which may not intuitively be a desired outcome in for example cancer treatment, is, however, emerging as an effective alternative strategy as compared to the aim of completely obliterating all vessels in the tumor. Especially when combined with cytotoxic agents, or radiation therapy, both of which require efficient

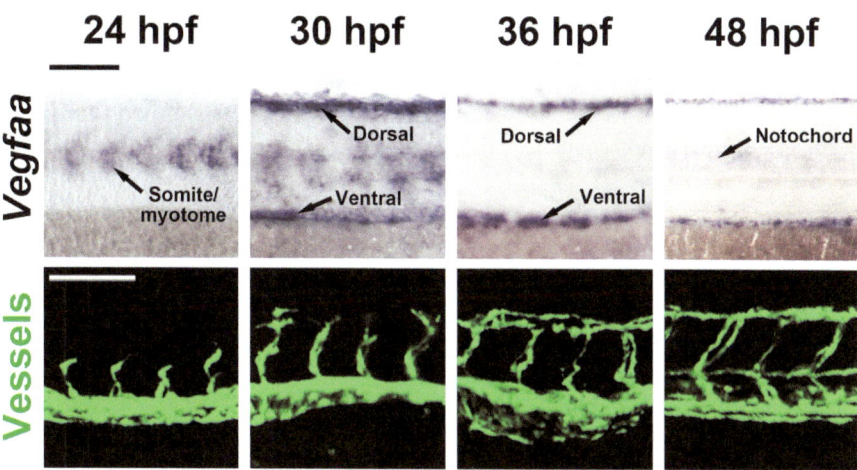

Fig. 1.4 Spatiotemporal expression of VEGF-A drives vascular patterning in zebrafish embryos. In situ hybridization showing *Vegfaa* mRNA expression in zebrafish embryos at 24–48 hours post fertilization (hpf) is shown in purple in the top row. *Vegfaa* is initially expressed in the myotomes but gradually relocate to the dorsal roof and ventral floor of the trunk at 36 hpf. At 48 hpf expression emerges in the notochord. These changes in expression correlate with areas of ongoing angiogenesis as shown in the lower row. Blood vessels of Tg(fli1a:EGFP)^{y1} zebrafish embryos shown in green start sprouting towards the VEGF-A signal at 24 h. At 36 h when *Vegfaa* expression has shifted to the dorsal roof of the trunk, formation of new sprouts leading to the construction of the dorsal-lateral anastomosing vessel in this site, takes place. At 48 hpf when notochord-expression is initiated, lymphatic progenitors sprout and form the transient parachordal lymphatic vessels. The *white* or *black* size bars indicate 100 µm

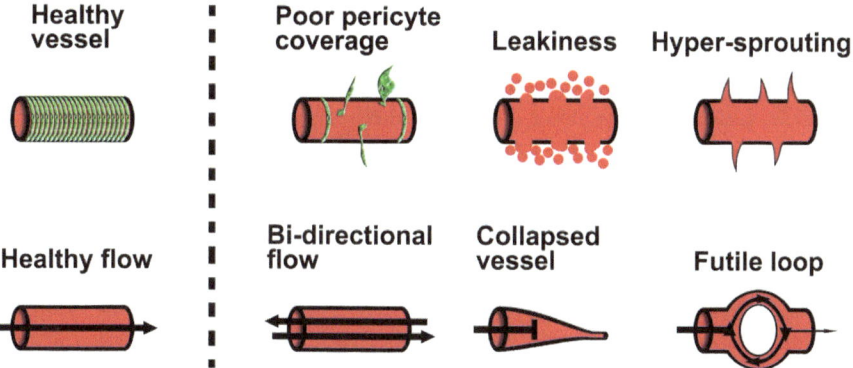

Fig. 1.5 Pathological phenotypes of blood vessels. In healthy tissues most capillaries (shown in *red*) are covered with pericytes (shown in *green*; *top-left image*), are relatively non-leaky, quiescent and exhibit uni-directional blood flow (*lower-left image*). In pathological conditions, however, pericyte coverage is diminished, vessels start leaking plasma into the tissue and non-directional hyper-sprouting as a part of ongoing angiogenesis is apparent (*top row*). Perfusion is also impaired as vessels may support flow in both directions (lack of arterial-venous identity), are often collapsed and non-perfused, or develop futile loops which do not support efficient perfusion through the tissue (*lower row*)

perfusion for maximal effects, such vascular maturation therapy might act synergistically to inhibit tumor growth rate (or even induce tumor regression) and importantly make the disease manageable compared to high-dose anti-angiogenic therapy which might lead to reduced effect of other treatment and could potentially even accelerate progression to metastatic disease, a risk that is intimately association with tumor hypoxia.

Lymphangiogenesis and Lymphatic Specification

Arteries and capillaries in healthy tissues are generally slightly leaky, which is the main mechanism of interstitial fluid production. Interstitial fluid, proteins, cellular and other types of debris is in turn collected by lymphatic vessels, a special vasculature that functions as the "sewage system" of the organism. The movement of fluid from arteries and capillaries to lymphatics is, however, also important for efficient delivery of nutrients and other factors through the tissues. The lymphatic vessels move the collected liquid and materials through an entirely afferent system, the content of which is eventually emptied into the cardinal vein at the duct of Cuvier, thereby transporting the liquid back into the blood from where it came. As such, the lymphatic vessels are essential for liquid homeostasis in the tissue and inefficient lymphatic functions or defective lymphatic developmental syndromes are primarily characterized by an accumulation of fluids (i.e. edema) [118]. As the interstitial fluid is rich in foreign proteins at sites of infection, the lymph (liquid in the lymphatic vessels) is first moved through the lymph nodes, where it bathes resident antigen-presenting dendritic cells, which in turn activate T- and B-cell responses against the invading pathogens. As such, lymph nodes both contribute to interstitial fluid drainage as well as adaptive immunity through being an integral component of the lymphatic system.

The lymphatic vessels are structurally and histologically different from blood vessels. Lymphatic capillaries emerge in blind-ended sacs in which the interstitial fluids are collected. As flow can only occur in one direction, the liquids will constantly be removed from the sacs, leading to a negative pressure which enables efficient "suction" and thus drainage of fluids [119]. The lymphatic endothelial cells in the capillary region has discontinuous and patchy basement membrane, which is not in direct contact with the lymphatic endothelial cells but rather is connected via filaments rendering the lymphatic endothelium naked. Furthermore, the lymphatic endothelial cells have no tight junctions but overlap one another in structures that function as valves only allowing liquid and macromolecules, cellular components or whole cells to flow in, but not out of the vessels. Just as in large veins, there are also valves in the lumens of the lymphatic vessels, which secure directional flow important for maintaining the negative pressure in the lymphatic sacs. Lymphatic capillaries drain into larger collecting lymphatic vessels, which are covered with smooth muscle cells that aid in the transport of lymph towards the lymph nodes and later the ducts of Cuvier [120]. The special structure of the lymphatic vessels is mirrored by a specific profile of genes being expressed in these vessels, which provide means to distinguish lymphatic vessels from blood vessels. The VEGF receptor three is a frequently used lymphatic-specific marker [26], although it has recently been found expressed also by tip cells in actively expanding blood vessels. However, as the lymphatic vessels are morphologically very different from tip cells, it is still convenient to use VEGFR3 staining as a histological tool. Lymphatic but not blood vessel endothelial cells also express the membrane glycoprotein LYVE-1, the transcription factor responsible for lymphatic endothelial identify, Prox1 and the adhesion protein Podoplanin [121, 122].

The main growth factor responsible for lymphatic vascular development and growth in adults is VEGF-C, which act primarily through VEGFR3 [123, 124]. During development, the induction of Prox-1 signaling in a sub-population of venous endothelial cells lead to the expression of VEGFR3 which in turn react to the secretion of VEGF-C by near-by arterial endothelial cells leading to the budding off and migration of these prox-1/vegfr3 positive lymphatic endothelial progenitors towards the VEGF-C source [122, 124]. The lymphatic endothelial cells aggregate as small lymphatic sacs or islands, which undergo morphologic transformation into the first lymphatic vessel, the thoracic duct, which connect to the cardinal vein only at the ducts of cuvier [123]. Other peripheral , posterior lymphatic vessels eventually grow by sprouting lymphangiogenesis from the thoracic duct, whereas anterior lymphatics in the head region of the embryo form by lymphvasculogenesis in a similar way as the thoracic duct is formed, and constitute the basis for expansion of the anterior lymphatic systems [125]. Under pathological conditions, however, inflammatory cytokines such as TNF-alpha are also potent lymphangiogenic signals, as recently identified in a corneal micropocket lymphangiogenesis model [26].

Concluding Remarks

In this chapter we have discussed how blood vessels are essential for the maintenance, development and differentiation, growth, regeneration and homeostasis of all tissues not only by serving as a transportation system for delivery of oxygen, nutrients and growth factors/other endocrine cytokines but also by forming niches through direct interaction with the cells in the tissues. The blood vessels have co-developed with the tissue and all capillary beds exhibit specific characteristics defined by the functions and needs of the tissue they exist in, respond to different growth factors in a tissue-specific manner and have different structure and density in for example the skeletal muscle, skin, adipose tissue, liver and central nervous system. The central mediators of vascular development and growth are members of the VEGF and VEGF receptor families with VEGF-A being generally important for the vascularization of most tissues, often in a hypoxia-dependent manner, and VEGF-C being of particular importance for lymphatic vessels. The vessels generally grow by sprouting angiogenesis a process which requires degradation of extracellular matrix, dissociation of perivascular cells, sprouting, longitudinal growth of the new vessel, anastomosis and lumen formation followed by maturation of the new vessel. This process is de-regulated under pathological conditions causing vessels to (1) grow in a non-directional manner, (2) anastomose and re-initiate sprouting prematurely and excessively leading to supraphysiological vascular density paradoxically coupled to hypoperfusion as a consequence of the formation of futile circulatory loops and blind-ended blood vessels, (3) inhibit pruning/degeneration of surplus vessels and increasing non-beneficial endothelial survival, (4) inhibit the development of the vascular wall and increase fenestration leading to high leakiness of the vessels, elevated interstitial fluid pressure and hemorrhaging and (5) are in many cases collapsed and non-perfused (summarized in Fig. 1.5). These characteristics of pathological vessels cause maintained or even increased tissue hypoxia, inflammation and therefore maintain the pathological state of the tissue [114].

Positive and negative regulation of blood vessel growth has proven a very challenging objective of medical intervention. While pathological growth of blood vessels in the eye, a prominent feature of diabetic retinopathy and age-related macular degeneration can be in many cases effectively treated by anti-VEGF-A therapy, leading to regained vision in nearly blind patients, the effects are in most cases not permanent and the vessels will eventually grow back and when they do they are refractive to anti-VEGF-A therapy [126, 127]. In cancer, however, the initially promising results from anti-VEGF-A therapy have faded. As the amount of patients treated with these drugs increased it became clear that problems with toxicity following prolonged systemic treatment, poor long-term efficacy due to resistance and possibly problematic treatment schedules leading to rapid neovascularization during drug holidays lead to poor if any overall survival benefit in treated patients [128]. As such, anti-VEGF-A treatment has now largely disappeared from the oncology clinics where such treatment is only used in a few indications such as glioblastoma, renal and colorectal cancer. It has thus become clear that pathological blood vessel growth is not dependent on a single factor, such as VEGF-A, but rather is the result of a multitude of pro-angiogenic signaling, and that the exact composition of such pro-angiogenic cocktails in pathological tissues is most likely context dependent and may differ from one patient to another [33, 128]. Even in eye disease, some patients are non-responsive to anti-VEGF treatment whereas others respond almost completely [126, 127], but angiogenesis is generally inhibited more effectively by broad and non-specific anti-inflammatory agents such as steroid-treatment [111]. This indicates that also in the context of a non-genetic and phenotypically rather homogeneous indication such as for example age-related macular degeneration, diabetic retinopathy or corneal neovascularization, single-target treatments are not likely to be effective in all patients. Broader-acting treatments or multiple single-target treatments should therefore be developed to effectively treat a larger group of cancer or retinopathy patients in the future. Conversely, pro-angiogenic stimulation as a strategy to combat ischemic diseases such as myocardial infarction, stroke or non-healing, ulcerating wounds, is a highly promising approach but also seem to rely on more than a single angiogenic factor. As such, despite promising results in pre-clinical models, the application of VEGF-A to sites of ischemic injury did not lead to the formation of a functional and mature vasculature but rather induced the rapid growth of "pathological" vessels which caused edema and were unstable [129]. Combinations of growth factors such as FGF-2 and PDGF-B or

HGF seem to be a more promising approach [13, 21], but results from clinical trials based on such strategies are still to be reported. Therapeutic lymphangiogenesis may also hold great potential for alleviating pathological edema in ischemic tissues, for example following myocardial infarction [130]. Recently it was discovered that angiogenesis may also be differentially regulated during the day and night [131, 132], indicating that circadian treatment schedules could be warranted. Furthermore, the angiogenic endothelial cells were reported to exhibit a different metabolism than quiescent endothelial cells, providing an additional target for anti-angiogenic therapy [133]. These findings still require further validation and the mechanisms needs to be more thoroughly characterized, but demonstrate that we still have much to learn about the regulation of angiogenesis and how this process may be targeted either positively or negatively in medicine.

References

1. Carmeliet P. Angiogenesis in health and disease. Nat Med. 2003;9:653–60.
2. Cao Y, Arbiser J, D'Amato RJ, D'Amore PA, Ingber DE, Kerbel R, Klagsbrun M, Lim S, Moses MA, Zetter B, Dvorak H, Langer R. Forty-year journey of angiogenesis translational research. Sci Transl Med. 2011;3:114rv113.
3. Crivellato E, Ribatti D. Aristotle: the first student of angiogenesis. Leukemia. 2006;20: 1209–10.
4. Natale G, Bocci G, Lenzi P. Looking for the word "angiogenesis" in the history of health sciences: from ancient times to the first decades of the twentieth century. World J Surg. 2016. doi:10.1007/s00268-016-3680-1
5. Cimpean AM, Ribatti D, Raica M. A brief history of angiogenesis assays. Int J Dev Biol. 2011;55:377–82.
6. Ferrara N, Henzel WJ. Pituitary follicular cells secrete a novel heparin-binding growth factor specific for vascular endothelial cells. Biochem Biophys Res Commun. 1989;161:851–8.
7. Gospodarowicz D, Abraham JA, Schilling J. Isolation and characterization of a vascular endothelial cell mitogen produced by pituitary-derived folliculo stellate cells. Proc Natl Acad Sci U S A. 1989;86:7311–5.
8. Vaisman N, Gospodarowicz D, Neufeld G. Characterization of the receptors for vascular endothelial growth factor. J Biol Chem. 1990;265:19461–6.
9. Plouet J, Moukadiri H. Characterization of the receptor to vasculotropin on bovine adrenal cortex-derived capillary endothelial cells. J Biol Chem. 1990;265:22071–4.
10. de Vries C, Escobedo JA, Ueno H, Houck K, Ferrara N, Williams LT. The fms-like tyrosine kinase, a receptor for vascular endothelial growth factor. Science. 1992;255:989–91.
11. Terman BI, Dougher-Vermazen M, Carrion ME, Dimitrov D, Armellino DC, Gospodarowicz D, Bohlen P. Identification of the KDR tyrosine kinase as a receptor for vascular endothelial cell growth factor. Biochem Biophys Res Commun. 1992;187:1579–86.
12. Zhang ZG, Zhang L, Jiang Q, Zhang R, Davies K, Powers C, Bruggen N, Chopp M. VEGF enhances angiogenesis and promotes blood-brain barrier leakage in the ischemic brain. J Clin Invest. 2000;106:829–38.
13. Banquet S, Gomez E, Nicol L, Edwards-Levy F, Henry JP, Cao R, Schapman D, Dautreaux B, Lallemand F, Bauer F, Cao Y, Thuillez C, Mulder P, Richard V, Brakenhielm E. Arteriogenic therapy by intramyocardial sustained delivery of a novel growth factor combination prevents chronic heart failure. Circulation. 2011;124:1059–69.
14. Cao Y. Adipose tissue angiogenesis as a therapeutic target for obesity and metabolic diseases. Nat Rev Drug Discov. 2010;9:107–15.

15. Gustafsson T, Kraus WE. Exercise-induced angiogenesis-related growth and transcription factors in skeletal muscle, and their modification in muscle pathology. Front Biosci. 2001;6:D75–89.
16. Folkman J. Tumor angiogenesis: therapeutic implications. N Engl J Med. 1971;285:1182–6.
17. Carmeliet P, Ferreira V, Breier G, Pollefeyt S, Kieckens L, Gertsenstein M, Fahrig M, Vandenhoeck A, Harpal K, Eberhardt C, Declercq C, Pawling J, Moons L, Collen D, Risau W, Nagy A. Abnormal blood vessel development and lethality in embryos lacking a single VEGF allele. Nature. 1996;380:435–9.
18. Gerhardt H, Golding M, Fruttiger M, Ruhrberg C, Lundkvist A, Abramsson A, Jeltsch M, Mitchell C, Alitalo K, Shima D, Betsholtz C. VEGF guides angiogenic sprouting utilizing endothelial tip cell filopodia. J Cell Biol. 2003;161:1163–77.
19. Jensen LD, Nakamura M, Brautigam L, Li X, Liu Y, Samani NJ, Cao Y. VEGF-B-Neuropilin-1 signaling is spatiotemporally indispensable for vascular and neuronal development in zebrafish. Proc Natl Acad Sci U S A. 2015;112:E5944–53.
20. Risau W. Mechanisms of angiogenesis. Nature. 1997;386:671–4.
21. Cao R, Brakenhielm E, Pawliuk R, Wariaro D, Post MJ, Wahlberg E, Leboulch P, Cao Y. Angiogenic synergism, vascular stability and improvement of hind-limb ischemia by a combination of PDGF-BB and FGF-2. Nat Med. 2003;9:604–13.
22. Cao R, Ji H, Yang Y, Cao Y. Collaborative effects between the TNFalpha-TNFR1-macrophage axis and the VEGF-C-VEGFR3 signaling in lymphangiogenesis and metastasis. Oncoimmunol. 2015;4:e989777.
23. Cao R, Ji H, Feng N, Zhang Y, Yang X, Andersson P, Sun Y, Tritsaris K, Hansen AJ, Dissing S, Cao Y. Collaborative interplay between FGF-2 and VEGF-C promotes lymphangiogenesis and metastasis. Proc Natl Acad Sci U S A. 2012;109:15894–9.
24. Cao R, Bjorndahl MA, Religa P, Clasper S, Garvin S, Galter D, Meister B, Ikomi F, Tritsaris K, Dissing S, Ohhashi T, Jackson DG, Cao Y. PDGF-BB induces intratumoral lymphangiogenesis and promotes lymphatic metastasis. Cancer Cell. 2004;6:333–45.
25. Nissen LJ, Cao R, Hedlund EM, Wang Z, Zhao X, Wetterskog D, Funa K, Brakenhielm E, Cao Y. Angiogenic factors FGF2 and PDGF-BB synergistically promote murine tumor neovascularization and metastasis. J Clin Invest. 2007;117:2766–77.
26. Ji H, Cao R, Yang Y, Zhang Y, Iwamoto H, Lim S, Nakamura M, Andersson P, Wang J, Sun Y, Dissing S, He X, Yang X, Cao Y. TNFR1 mediates TNF-alpha-induced tumour lymphangiogenesis and metastasis by modulating VEGF-C-VEGFR3 signalling. Nat Commun. 2014;5:4944.
27. Ueki N, Nakazato M, Ohkawa T, Ikeda T, Amuro Y, Hada T, Higashino K. Excessive production of transforming growth-factor beta 1 can play an important role in the development of tumorigenesis by its action for angiogenesis: validity of neutralizing antibodies to block tumor growth. Biochim Biophys Acta. 1992;1137:189–96.
28. Pan B, Shen J, Cao J, Zhou Y, Shang L, Jin S, Cao S, Che D, Liu F, Yu Y. Interleukin-17 promotes angiogenesis by stimulating VEGF production of cancer cells via the STAT3/GIV signaling pathway in non-small-cell lung cancer. Sci Report. 2015;5:16053.
29. Wang J, Wang Y, Wang S, Cai J, Shi J, Sui X, Cao Y, Huang W, Chen X, Cai Z, Li H, Bardeesi AS, Zhang B, Liu M, Song W, Wang M, Xiang AP. Bone marrow-derived mesenchymal stem cell-secreted IL-8 promotes the angiogenesis and growth of colorectal cancer. Oncotarget. 2015;6:42825–37.
30. Yang Y, Andersson P, Hosaka K, Zhang Y, Cao R, Iwamoto H, Yang X, Nakamura M, Wang J, Zhuang R, Morikawa H, Xue Y, Braun H, Beyaert R, Samani N, Nakae S, Hams E, Dissing S, Fallon PG, Langer R, Cao Y. The PDGF-BB-SOX7 axis-modulated IL-33 in pericytes and stromal cells promotes metastasis through tumour-associated macrophages. Nat Commun. 2016;7:11385.
31. Ferrara N. Role of myeloid cells in vascular endothelial growth factor-independent tumor angiogenesis. Curr Opin Hematol. 2010;17:219–24.
32. Lu P, Weaver VM, Werb Z. The extracellular matrix: a dynamic niche in cancer progression. J Cell Biol. 2012;196:395–406.

33. Cao Y. Opinion: emerging mechanisms of tumour lymphangiogenesis and lymphatic metastasis. Nat Rev Cancer. 2005;5:735–43.

34. Vanhollebeke B, Stone OA, Bostaille N, Cho C, Zhou Y, Maquet E, Gauquier A, Cabochette P, Fukuhara S, Mochizuki N, Nathans J, Stainier DY. Tip cell-specific requirement for an atypical Gpr124- and Reck-dependent Wnt/beta-catenin pathway during brain angiogenesis. Elife. 2015;4:e06489.

35. Zhou Y, Nathans J. Gpr124 controls CNS angiogenesis and blood-brain barrier integrity by promoting ligand-specific canonical wnt signaling. Dev Cell. 2014;31:248–56.

36. Cao R, Brakenhielm E, Wahlestedt C, Thyberg J, Cao Y. Leptin induces vascular permeability and synergistically stimulates angiogenesis with FGF-2 and VEGF. Proc Natl Acad Sci U S A. 2001;98:6390–5.

37. Brakenhielm E, Cao R, Gao B, Angelin B, Cannon B, Parini P, Cao Y. Angiogenesis inhibitor, TNP-470, prevents diet-induced and genetic obesity in mice. Circ Res. 2004;94:1579–88.

38. Xue Y, Petrovic N, Cao R, Larsson O, Lim S, Chen S, Feldmann HM, Liang Z, Zhu Z, Nedergaard J, Cannon B, Cao Y. Hypoxia-independent angiogenesis in adipose tissues during cold acclimation. Cell Metab. 2009;9:99–109.

39. Thomas PR, Nash GB, Dormandy JA. White cell accumulation in dependent legs of patients with venous hypertension: a possible mechanism for trophic changes in the skin. Br Med J (Clin Res Ed). 1988;296:1693–5.

40. Kwong KK, Belliveau JW, Chesler DA, Goldberg IE, Weisskoff RM, Poncelet BP, Kennedy DN, Hoppel BE, Cohen MS, Turner R, et al. Dynamic magnetic resonance imaging of human brain activity during primary sensory stimulation. Proc Natl Acad Sci U S A. 1992;89:5675–9.

41. Stacy MR, Caracciolo CM, Qiu M, Pal P, Varga T, Constable RT, Sinusas AJ. Comparison of regional skeletal muscle tissue oxygenation in college athletes and sedentary control subjects using quantitative BOLD MR imaging. Phys Rep. 2016;4:1–10. doi:10.14814/phy2.12903

42. Iadecola C, Nedergaard M. Glial regulation of the cerebral microvasculature. Nat Neurosci. 2007;10:1369–76.

43. Wei HS, Kang H, Rasheed IY, Zhou S, Lou N, Gershteyn A, McConnell ED, Wang Y, Richardson KE, Palmer AF, Xu C, Wan J, Nedergaard M. Erythrocytes are oxygen-sensing regulators of the cerebral microcirculation. Neuron. 2016;91:851–62.

44. During MJ, Liu X, Huang W, Magee D, Slater A, McMurphy T, Wang C, Cao L. Adipose VEGF links the white-to-brown fat switch with environmental, genetic, and pharmacological stimuli in male mice. Endocrinology. 2015;156:2059–73.

45. Cao Y. Angiogenesis and vascular functions in modulation of obesity, adipose metabolism, and insulin sensitivity. Cell Metab. 2013;18:478–89.

46. Xue Y, Cao R, Nilsson D, Chen S, Westergren R, Hedlund EM, Martijn C, Rondahl L, Krauli P, Walum E, Enerback S, Cao Y. FOXC2 controls Ang-2 expression and modulates angiogenesis, vascular patterning, remodeling, and functions in adipose tissue. Proc Natl Acad Sci U S A. 2008;105:10167–72.

47. McCall AL, van Bueren AM, Huang L, Stenbit A, Celnik E, Charron MJ. Forebrain endothelium expresses GLUT4, the insulin-responsive glucose transporter. Brain Res. 1997;744:318–26.

48. Stenman JM, Rajagopal J, Carroll TJ, Ishibashi M, McMahon J, McMahon AP. Canonical Wnt signaling regulates organ-specific assembly and differentiation of CNS vasculature. Science. 2008;322:1247–50.

49. Scholzen TE, Brzoska T, Kalden DH, Hartmeyer M, Fastrich M, Luger TA, Armstrong CA, Ansel JC. Expression of functional melanocortin receptors and proopiomelanocortin peptides by human dermal microvascular endothelial cells. Ann N Y Acad Sci. 1999;885:239–53.

50. Russell KS, Haynes MP, Sinha D, Clerisme E, Bender JR. Human vascular endothelial cells contain membrane binding sites for estradiol, which mediate rapid intracellular signaling. Proc Natl Acad Sci U S A. 2000;97:5930–5.

51. Reiss Y, Engelhardt B. T cell interaction with ICAM-1-deficient endothelium in vitro: transendothelial migration of different T cell populations is mediated by endothelial ICAM-1 and ICAM-2. Int Immunol. 1999;11:1527–39.

52. Gonzalez-Alonso J. Human thermoregulation and the cardiovascular system. Exp Physiol. 2012;97:340–6.
53. Daanen HA, Van Marken Lichtenbelt WD. Human whole body cold adaptation. Temperature (Austin). 2016;3:104–18.
54. Gerhart-Hines Z, Feng D, Emmett MJ, Everett LJ, Loro E, Briggs ER, Bugge A, Hou C, Ferrara C, Seale P, Pryma DA, Khurana TS, Lazar MA. The nuclear receptor Rev-erbalpha controls circadian thermogenic plasticity. Nature. 2013;503:410–3.
55. Scadden DT. The stem-cell niche as an entity of action. Nature. 2006;441:1075–9.
56. Ottone C, Krusche B, Whitby A, Clements M, Quadrato G, Pitulescu ME, Adams RH, Parrinello S. Direct cell-cell contact with the vascular niche maintains quiescent neural stem cells. Nat Cell Biol. 2014;16:1045–56.
57. Gomez-Gaviro MV, Lovell-Badge R, Fernandez-Aviles F, Lara-Pezzi E. The vascular stem cell niche. J Cardiovasc Transl Res. 2012;5:618–30.
58. Gupta RK, Mepani RJ, Kleiner S, Lo JC, Khandekar MJ, Cohen P, Frontini A, Bhowmick DC, Ye L, Cinti S, Spiegelman BM. Zfp423 expression identifies committed preadipocytes and localizes to adipose endothelial and perivascular cells. Cell Metab. 2012;15:230–9.
59. Hughes R, Qian BZ, Rowan C, Muthana M, Keklikoglou I, Olson OC, Tazzyman S, Danson S, Addison C, Clemons M, Gonzalez-Angulo AM, Joyce JA, De Palma M, Pollard JW, Lewis CE. Perivascular M2 macrophages stimulate tumor relapse after chemotherapy. Cancer Res. 2015;75:3479–91.
60. Hislop AA. Airway and blood vessel interaction during lung development. J Anat. 2002;201:325–34.
61. Sequeira Lopez ML, Gomez RA. Development of the renal arterioles. J Am Soc Nephrol. 2011;22:2156–65.
62. Si-Tayeb K, Lemaigre FP, Duncan SA. Organogenesis and development of the liver. Dev Cell. 2010;18:175–89.
63. Ekstrand AJ, Cao R, Bjorndahl M, Nystrom S, Jonsson-Rylander AC, Hassani H, Hallberg B, Nordlander M, Cao Y. Deletion of neuropeptide Y (NPY) 2 receptor in mice results in blockage of NPY-induced angiogenesis and delayed wound healing. Proc Natl Acad Sci U S A. 2003;100:6033–8.
64. Alvarez Y, Astudillo O, Jensen L, Reynolds AL, Waghorne N, Brazil DP, Cao Y, O'Connor JJ, Kennedy BN. Selective inhibition of retinal angiogenesis by targeting PI3 kinase. PLoS One. 2009;4:e7867.
65. Korzh S, Pan X, Garcia-Lecea M, Winata CL, Pan X, Wohland T, Korzh V, Gong Z. Requirement of vasculogenesis and blood circulation in late stages of liver growth in zebrafish. BMC Dev Biol. 2008;8:84.
66. Majumdar A, Drummond IA. Podocyte differentiation in the absence of endothelial cells as revealed in the zebrafish avascular mutant, cloche. Dev Genet. 1999;24:220–9.
67. Paulsson M. Basement membrane proteins: structure, assembly, and cellular interactions. Crit Rev Biochem Mol Biol. 1992;27:93–127.
68. Zhang Y, Yang Y, Hosaka K, Huang G, Zang J, Chen F, Zhang Y, Samani NJ, Cao Y. Endocrine vasculatures are preferable targets of an antitumor ineffective low dose of anti-VEGF therapy. Proc Natl Acad Sci U S A. 2016;113:4158–63.
69. Birbrair A, Zhang T, Files DC, Mannava S, Smith T, Wang ZM, Messi ML, Mintz A, Delbono O. Type-1 pericytes accumulate after tissue injury and produce collagen in an organ-dependent manner. Stem Cell Res Ther. 2014;5:122.
70. Birbrair A, Zhang T, Wang ZM, Messi ML, Mintz A, Delbono O. Pericytes at the intersection between tissue regeneration and pathology. Clin Sci (Lond). 2015;128:81–93.
71. Geevarghese A, Herman IM. Pericyte-endothelial crosstalk: implications and opportunities for advanced cellular therapies. Transl Res. 2014;163:296–306.
72. Dahl Ejby Jensen L, Cao R, Hedlund EM, Soll I, Lundberg JO, Hauptmann G, Steffensen JF, Cao Y. Nitric oxide permits hypoxia-induced lymphatic perfusion by controlling arterial-lymphatic conduits in zebrafish and glass catfish. Proc Natl Acad Sci U S A. 2009;106: 18408–13.

73. Jensen LD, Rouhi P, Cao Z, Lanne T, Wahlberg E, Cao Y. Zebrafish models to study hypoxia-induced pathological angiogenesis in malignant and nonmalignant diseases. Birth Defects Res C Embryo Today. 2011;93:182–93.
74. Gordan R, Gwathmey JK, Xie LH. Autonomic and endocrine control of cardiovascular function. World J Cardiol. 2015;7:204–14.
75. Ricciotti E, FitzGerald GA. Prostaglandins and inflammation. Arterioscler Thromb Vasc Biol. 2011;31:986–1000.
76. Keith IM. The role of endogenous lung neuropeptides in regulation of the pulmonary circulation. Physiol Res. 2000;49:519–37.
77. Heil M, Schaper W. Influence of mechanical, cellular, and molecular factors on collateral artery growth (arteriogenesis). Circ Res. 2004;95:449–58.
78. Galie PA, Nguyen DH, Choi CK, Cohen DM, Janmey PA, Chen CS. Fluid shear stress threshold regulates angiogenic sprouting. Proc Natl Acad Sci U S A. 2014;111:7968–73.
79. Nicoli S, Standley C, Walker P, Hurlstone A, Fogarty KE, Lawson ND. MicroRNA-mediated integration of haemodynamics and Vegf signalling during angiogenesis. Nature. 2010;464:1196–200.
80. Lawson ND, Vogel AM, Weinstein BM. sonic hedgehog and vascular endothelial growth factor act upstream of the Notch pathway during arterial endothelial differentiation. Dev Cell. 2002;3:127–36.
81. Gore AV, Monzo K, Cha YR, Pan W, Weinstein BM. Vascular development in the zebrafish. Cold Spring Harb Perspect Med. 2012;2:a006684.
82. Kamei M, Saunders WB, Bayless KJ, Dye L, Davis GE, Weinstein BM. Endothelial tubes assemble from intracellular vacuoles in vivo. Nature. 2006;442:453–6.
83. Lammert E, Axnick J. Vascular lumen formation. Cold Spring Harb Perspect Med. 2012;2:a006619.
84. Gritz E, Hirschi KK. Specification and function of hemogenic endothelium during embryogenesis. Cell Mol Life Sci. 2016;73:1547–67.
85. Herbert SP, Huisken J, Kim TN, Feldman ME, Houseman BT, Wang RA, Shokat KM, Stainier DY. Arterial-venous segregation by selective cell sprouting: an alternative mode of blood vessel formation. Science. 2009;326:294–8.
86. Isogai S, Horiguchi M, Weinstein BM. The vascular anatomy of the developing zebrafish: an atlas of embryonic and early larval development. Dev Biol. 2001;230:278–301.
87. Rundhaug JE. Matrix metalloproteinases and angiogenesis. J Cell Mol Med. 2005;9:267–85.
88. Siekmann AF, Lawson ND. Notch signalling limits angiogenic cell behaviour in developing zebrafish arteries. Nature. 2007;445:781–4.
89. Hellstrom M, Phng LK, Hofmann JJ, Wallgard E, Coultas L, Lindblom P, Alva J, Nilsson AK, Karlsson L, Gaiano N, Yoon K, Rossant J, Iruela-Arispe ML, Kalen M, Gerhardt H, Betsholtz C. Dll4 signalling through Notch1 regulates formation of tip cells during angiogenesis. Nature. 2007;445:776–80.
90. Cao R, Jensen LD, Soll I, Hauptmann G, Cao Y. Hypoxia-induced retinal angiogenesis in zebrafish as a model to study retinopathy. PLoS One. 2008;3:e2748.
91. Jakobsson L, Franco CA, Bentley K, Collins RT, Ponsioen B, Aspalter IM, Rosewell I, Busse M, Thurston G, Medvinsky A, Schulte-Merker S, Gerhardt H. Endothelial cells dynamically compete for the tip cell position during angiogenic sprouting. Nat Cell Biol. 2010;12:943–53.
92. Herwig L, Blum Y, Krudewig A, Ellertsdottir E, Lenard A, Belting HG, Affolter M. Distinct cellular mechanisms of blood vessel fusion in the zebrafish embryo. Curr Biol. 2011;21:1942–8.
93. Fantin A, Vieira JM, Gestri G, Denti L, Schwarz Q, Prykhozhij S, Peri F, Wilson SW, Ruhrberg C. Tissue macrophages act as cellular chaperones for vascular anastomosis downstream of VEGF-mediated endothelial tip cell induction. Blood. 2010;116:829–40.
94. Lindblom P, Gerhardt H, Liebner S, Abramsson A, Enge M, Hellstrom M, Backstrom G, Fredriksson S, Landegren U, Nystrom HC, Bergstrom G, Dejana E, Ostman A, Lindahl P,

Betsholtz C. Endothelial PDGF-B retention is required for proper investment of pericytes in the microvessel wall. Genes Dev. 2003;17:1835–40.

95. Krueger J, Liu D, Scholz K, Zimmer A, Shi Y, Klein C, Siekmann A, Schulte-Merker S, Cudmore M, Ahmed A, le Noble F. Flt1 acts as a negative regulator of tip cell formation and branching morphogenesis in the zebrafish embryo. Development. 2011;138:2111–20.
96. Lamalice L, Le Boeuf F, Huot J. Endothelial cell migration during angiogenesis. Circ Res. 2007;100:782–94.
97. Adams RH, Eichmann A. Axon guidance molecules in vascular patterning. Cold Spring Harb Perspect Biol. 2010;2:a001875.
98. Torres-Vazquez J, Gitler AD, Fraser SD, Berk JD, Van NP, Fishman MC, Childs S, Epstein JA, Weinstein BM. Semaphorin-plexin signaling guides patterning of the developing vasculature. Dev Cell. 2004;7:117–23.
99. Jung B, Obinata H, Galvani S, Mendelson K, Ding BS, Skoura A, Kinzel B, Brinkmann V, Rafii S, Evans T, Hla T. Flow-regulated endothelial S1P receptor-1 signaling sustains vascular development. Dev Cell. 2012;23:600–10.
100. Ribatti D, Nico B, Crivellato E. The role of pericytes in angiogenesis. Int J Dev Biol. 2011;55:261–8.
101. Burri PH, Djonov V. Intussusceptive angiogenesis--the alternative to capillary sprouting. Mol Asp Med. 2002;23:S1–27.
102. Gianni-Barrera R, Trani M, Fontanellaz C, Heberer M, Djonov V, Hlushchuk R, Banfi A. VEGF over-expression in skeletal muscle induces angiogenesis by intussusception rather than sprouting. Angiogenesis. 2013;16:123–36.
103. Dimova I, Hlushchuk R, Makanya A, Styp-Rekowska B, Ceausu A, Flueckiger S, Lang S, Semela D, Le Noble F, Chatterjee S, Djonov V. Inhibition of Notch signaling induces extensive intussusceptive neo-angiogenesis by recruitment of mononuclear cells. Angiogenesis. 2013;16:921–37.
104. Mukwaya A, Peebo B, Xeroudaki M, Ali Z, Lennikov A, Jensen L, Lagali N. Factors regulating capillary remodeling in a reversible model of inflammatory corneal angiogenesis. Sci Report. 2016;6:32137.
105. Djonov V, Schmid M, Tschanz SA, Burri PH. Intussusceptive angiogenesis: its role in embryonic vascular network formation. Circ Res. 2000;86:286–92.
106. Makanya AN, Hlushchuk R, Baum O, Velinov N, Ochs M, Djonov V. Microvascular endowment in the developing chicken embryo lung. Am J Phys Lung Cell Mol Phys. 2007;292:L1136–46.
107. Kilarski WW, Samolov B, Petersson L, Kvanta A, Gerwins P. Biomechanical regulation of blood vessel growth during tissue vascularization. Nat Med. 2009;15:657–64.
108. Huang CC, Lawson ND, Weinstein BM, Johnson SL. reg6 is required for branching morphogenesis during blood vessel regeneration in zebrafish caudal fins. Dev Biol. 2003;264:263–74.
109. Fruttiger M. Development of the retinal vasculature. Angiogenesis. 2007;10:77–88.
110. Lenard A, Daetwyler S, Betz C, Ellertsdottir E, Belting HG, Huisken J, Affolter M. Endothelial cell self-fusion during vascular pruning. PLoS Biol. 2015;13:e1002126.
111. Mirabelli P, Peebo BB, Xeroudaki M, Koulikovska M, Lagali N. Early effects of dexamethasone and anti-VEGF therapy in an inflammatory corneal neovascularization model. Exp Eye Res. 2014;125:118–27.
112. Mancuso MR, Davis R, Norberg SM, O'Brien S, Sennino B, Nakahara T, Yao VJ, Inai T, Brooks P, Freimark B, Shalinsky DR, Hu-Lowe DD, McDonald DM. Rapid vascular regrowth in tumors after reversal of VEGF inhibition. J Clin Invest. 2006;116:2610–21.
113. Noguera-Troise I, Daly C, Papadopoulos NJ, Coetzee S, Boland P, Gale NW, Lin HC, Yancopoulos GD, Thurston G. Blockade of Dll4 inhibits tumour growth by promoting nonproductive angiogenesis. Nature. 2006;444:1032–7.
114. Goel S, Duda DG, Xu L, Munn LL, Boucher Y, Fukumura D, Jain RK. Normalization of the vasculature for treatment of cancer and other diseases. Physiol Rev. 2011;91:1071–121.

115. Larrivee B, Freitas C, Trombe M, Lv X, Delafarge B, Yuan L, Bouvree K, Breant C, Del Toro R, Brechot N, Germain S, Bono F, Dol F, Claes F, Fischer C, Autiero M, Thomas JL, Carmeliet P, Tessier-Lavigne M, Eichmann A. Activation of the UNC5B receptor by Netrin-1 inhibits sprouting angiogenesis. Genes Dev. 2007;21: 2433–47.

116. Miloudi K, Binet F, Wilson A, Cerani A, Oubaha M, Menard C, Henriques S, Mawambo G, Dejda A, Nguyen PT, Rezende FA, Bourgault S, Kennedy TE, Sapieha P. Truncated netrin-1 contributes to pathological vascular permeability in diabetic retinopathy. J Clin Invest. 2016;126:3006–22.

117. Neufeld G, Sabag AD, Rabinovicz N, Kessler O. Semaphorins in angiogenesis and tumor progression. Cold Spring Harb Perspect Med. 2012;2:a006718.

118. Alders M, Hogan BM, Gjini E, Salehi F, Al-Gazali L, Hennekam EA, Holmberg EE, Mannens MM, Mulder MF, Offerhaus GJ, Prescott TE, Schroor EJ, Verheij JB, Witte M, Zwijnenburg PJ, Vikkula M, Schulte-Merker S, Hennekam RC. Mutations in CCBE1 cause generalized lymph vessel dysplasia in humans. Nat Genet. 2009;41:1272–4.

119. Munn LL. Mechanobiology of lymphatic contractions. Semin Cell Dev Biol. 2015;38:67–74.

120. Betterman KL, Paquet-Fifield S, Asselin-Labat ML, Visvader JE, Butler LM, Stacker SA, Achen MG, Harvey NL. Remodeling of the lymphatic vasculature during mouse mammary gland morphogenesis is mediated via epithelial-derived lymphangiogenic stimuli. Am J Pathol. 2012;181:2225–38.

121. Sironi M, Conti A, Bernasconi S, Fra AM, Pasqualini F, Nebuloni M, Lauri E, De Bortoli M, Mantovani A, Dejana E, Vecchi A. Generation and characterization of a mouse lymphatic endothelial cell line. Cell Tissue Res. 2006;325:91–100.

122. Wigle JT, Harvey N, Detmar M, Lagutina I, Grosveld G, Gunn MD, Jackson DG, Oliver G. An essential role for Prox1 in the induction of the lymphatic endothelial cell phenotype. EMBO J. 2002;21:1505–13.

123. Adams RH, Alitalo K. Molecular regulation of angiogenesis and lymphangiogenesis. Nat Rev Mol Cell Biol. 2007;8:464–78.

124. Karkkainen MJ, Haiko P, Sainio K, Partanen J, Taipale J, Petrova TV, Jeltsch M, Jackson DG, Talikka M, Rauvala H, Betsholtz C, Alitalo K. Vascular endothelial growth factor C is required for sprouting of the first lymphatic vessels from embryonic veins. Nat Immunol. 2004;5:74–80.

125. Okuda KS, Astin JW, Misa JP, Flores MV, Crosier KE, Crosier PS. lyve1 expression reveals novel lymphatic vessels and new mechanisms for lymphatic vessel development in zebrafish. Development. 2012;139:2381–91.

126. Yang S, Zhao J, Sun X. Resistance to anti-VEGF therapy in neovascular age-related macular degeneration: a comprehensive review. Drug Des Devel Ther. 2016;10:1857–67.

127. Yang Y, Bailey C, Holz FG, Eter N, Weber M, Baker C, Kiss S, Menchini U, Ruiz Moreno JM, Dugel P, Lotery A, FAME study group. Long-term outcomes of phakic patients with diabetic macular oedema treated with intravitreal fluocinolone acetonide (FAc) implants. Eye (Lond). 2015;29:1173–80.

128. Cao Y. Antiangiogenic cancer therapy: why do mouse and human patients respond in a different way to the same drug? Int J Dev Biol. 2011;55:557–62.

129. Cao Y. Therapeutic angiogenesis for ischemic disorders: what is missing for clinical benefits? Discov Med. 2010;9:179–84.

130. Henri O, Pouehe C, Houssari M, Galas L, Nicol L, Edwards-Levy F, Henry JP, Dumesnil A, Boukhalfa I, Banquet S, Schapman D, Thuillez C, Richard V, Mulder P, Brakenhielm E. Selective stimulation of cardiac lymphangiogenesis reduces myocardial edema and fibrosis leading to improved cardiac function following myocardial infarction. Circulation. 2016;133:1484–97; discussion 1497.

131. Jensen LD, Gyllenhaal C, Block K. Circadian angiogenesis. Biomol Concepts. 2014;5:245–56.

132. Jensen LD, Cao Z, Nakamura M, Yang Y, Brautigam L, Andersson P, Zhang Y, Wahlberg E, Lanne T, Hosaka K, Cao Y. Opposing effects of circadian clock genes bmal1 and period2 in regulation of VEGF-dependent angiogenesis in developing zebrafish. Cell Rep. 2012;2:231–41.
133. Cruys B, Wong BW, Kuchnio A, Verdegem D, Cantelmo AR, Conradi LC, Vandekeere S, Bouche A, Cornelissen I, Vinckier S, Merks RM, Dejana E, Gerhardt H, Dewerchin M, Bentley K, Carmeliet P. Glycolytic regulation of cell rearrangement in angiogenesis. Nat Commun. 2016;7:12240.

Infantile Hemangioma: New Insights on Pathogenesis and Beta Blockers Mechanisms of Action

Shoshana Greenberger

Introduction

Infantile hemangioma (IH) is the most common tumor of infancy, affecting 5–10% of infants at the end of the first year. Increased risk factors for IH include Caucasian race, female gender (4:1 female to male ratio) [1], prematurity, low birth weight, and being the product of multiple gestations [2]. There is increased risk in premature neonates under the weight of 1,500 g, in females and in Caucasians. The superficial tumors are usually noticed initially in the first 4 weeks after birth as brightly red macule, papule or plaque. In contrast, deep-seated IHs often present later, at 2–3 months of age, as soft blue nodules.

Clinical

IH is a benign tumor, and in most patients it carries no risk of morbidity or mortality. However, in 10% of patients IH is problematic or even endangering to the child, due to its anatomical location or due to excessive growth. The great majority of IH are focal and solitary. Sixty percent of the tumors occur on the head and neck, 25% on the trunk, and 15% on the extremities. The tumor displays a unique life cycle that can be separated clinically into three phases [3, 4]. The proliferating phase starts within first weeks of life and ends within the first year of life, with the most growth occurring during the first 4–6 months of life. At this phase, the tumor changes its presentation from mild blanching, fine telangiectasias or a red or macule to a prominent bright red papule, plaque or nodule [5]. The involution phase begins on average at 12 months of age. The tumor changes color from bright red to less red and gray. Also,

S. Greenberger
The Department of Dermatology and Sheba Cancer Research Center, Sheba Medical Center, Ramat-Gan 52621, Israel
e-mail: shoshana.greenberger@sheba.health.gov.il

© Springer-Verlag London Ltd. 2017
J.L. Arbiser (ed.), *Angiogenesis-Based Dermatology*,
DOI 10.1007/978-1-4471-7314-4_2

nodules and papules shrink and soften. Finally, at the involuted phase, tumor growth has stopped and the tumor regressed. About half of tumors involute by age 5 years and 70% by age 7 years. In 30%, an additional 3–5 years to complete the process [6]. The regression of IH often leaves residues. These residues are correlated to the maximum size of the hemangioma. These include telangiectasias, atrophic, wrinkled skin, hyper or hypopigmentation as well as redundant fibrofatty tissue [7].

Histopathology and Cellular Components

The pathological phases of IH strongly correlate with the clinical phases. The proliferating lesions display solid, cellular lobules consisting of plump endothelial cells lining tiny rounded vascular spaces with inconspicuous lumina. In the involuting phase the vascular channels contain flattened, mature, endothelial cells, an organized perivascular layer and basement membrane. Apoptotic cells, at least third of them endothelial are seen [8–10] and an increase in the number of mast cells. Lastly, at the involuted phase, fat, fibroblasts and connective tissue replace the vascular tissue, with few remaining large feeding and draining vessels evident.

In recent years, several cellular components of IH were isolated and characterized. These include hemangioma-derived progenitor/stem cells (HemSCs), endothelial progenitor cells (HemEPCs), ECs (HemECs) and perivascular cells (Hem-pericytes).

HemSC

The etiology of IH is still unknown. Over the years, several researchers speculated an aberrant embryonic developmental in situ or placental embolic origin of IH during early fetal life. The 'placental theory' is based on the co-expression of placental antigens, such as glucose transporter-1 (GLUT-1), merosin, Lewis Y antigen, FCγRIII, and type 3-iodothyronine deiodinase in IH ([11–13]). In addition, a higher incidence of IH has also been observed following amniocentesis and chorionic villous sampling (CVS) [14, 15]. Supporting the hypothesis of dysregulated embryonic differentiation is the identification of progenitor/stem cells in IH. In 2008 the Bischoff group isolated a primitive mesenchymal cell [16] using anti-CD133-coated magnetic beads. These rare cells, comprising 0.1–1% of the cells in proliferating phase IH have the ability to self-renew and undergo multi-lineage differentiation. Differently from Bone marrow mesenchymal progenitor cells, HemSC differentiate not only towards adipocytes, osteocytes and chondrocytes but also into endothelium. When implanted sub-cutaneously into immune-deficient mice, the HemSC form GLUT1+ vessels. Tracing the cells in vivo demonstrated that HemSC form the two layer of the capillaries- endothelium and pericytes [17]. Later, HemSC differentiate into adipocytes [16]. Other groups reported similar results. Xu et al. isolated stem cells from IH using selective culture media and grew tumor sphere that expressed CD133 and the progenitor cell marker SALL4. Injection into immunodeficient mice produced GLUT1 positive tumors [18].

Itinteang T et al. demonstrated the expression of embryonic stem cell (ESC) markers, Nanog, SALL4, and CD133 in the proliferative phase of IH with reduced expression during lesion involution [19, 20]. Taken together, these findings suggested that IH is not only a disorder of angiogenesis (i.e., the sprouting of new vessels from existing ones) but also a disorder of vasculogenesis (i.e., the de novo formation of new blood vessels from stem cells)

Endothelial Cells

Endothelial cells constitute about 30% of the proliferating tumor. Morphologically the cells are plump in the proliferating tumor and spindle shape in the involuting phase [21]. In vitro studies showed that both in terms of cell morphology and protein expression hemangioma endothelial cells are more characteristic of embryonic microvascular endothelial cells than that of postembryonic cells [8]. The cells express typical endothelial-specific markers such as von Willebrand Factor, CD31/PECAM-1, and E-selectin KDR, TIE-2, and VE-cadherin [22, 23]. In addition, North and colleagues showed that glucose transporter-1 (GLUT1) is expressed on hemangioma endothelium, whereas no expression is noted in other types of vascular tumors and vascular malformations [24]. Consequently GLUT1 became a useful diagnostic marker. HemEC were shown by Boye and colleagues to be clonal, suggesting they arise from a common precursor [22].

Hemangioma endothelial progenitor cells (HemEPC) are less differentiated cells that were isolated based on the human stem cell marker CD133. These cells constitute a small percentage (0.1–2%) of the total endothelial cells. HemEPC, similarly to HemEC, share properties with cord-blood endothelial colony–forming cells (CB-ECFCs) including paradoxical stimulation by endostatin, suggesting that the two cell types have immature phenotype [25, 26].

Myeloid Cells and Macrophages

The presence of myeloid cells in IH, and more specifically macrophages, have been shown in several studies [27, 28]. Macrophages perform phagocytic clearance of dying cells and protect the host through innate immunity, both as resident tissue macrophages and as monocyte-derived recruited cells during inflammation. Classically, macrophages have been divided into two types: The M1-polarised macrophages are activated by microbial antigens and respond to Th1 immune cells by the secretion of pro-inflammatory cytokines. The M2-polarized macrophages secrete anti-inflammatory pro-angiogenic factors in response to Th2 cells [29]. Both M1 and M2 Macrophages were shown to be more prevalent in proliferating IHs than in involuting lesions [27, 30], with M1 being more prevalent. The cells are located in the interstitium, between the vessels, and were shown to increase the proliferation of HemSC. In addition, conditioned media from either M1- or M2-polarized macrophages significantly suppressed the adipogenesis of HemSC [30]. Thus, macrophages may have a role in the proliferation of IH.

Pericytes

Pericytes are contractile mural cells that are located around the EC of capillaries and venules. The cells that can be distinguished from vascular smooth muscle cells by the expression of distinct set molecular markers including platelet-derived growth factor receptor β (PDGFRβ), CD146, aminopeptidases A and N (CD13), endoglin, neuron-glial 2 (NG2) [31–33]. Throughout the vasculature pericytes have a central role in endothelial barrier development and maintenance of integrity [34]. In addition, the microvascular tone is regulate, in large, by the pericytes [35].

In IH, pericytes are abundant in both the proliferating and the involuting phases [20]. In vitro and in vivo studies have shown that HemSC differentiate into pericytes upon direct contact with EC. Jagged-1, a Notch ligand, is required for the differentiation process [17]. Thus, the source of the pericytes in the tumor might be the HemSC. Boscolo et al. demonstrated that IH pericytes differ from normal pericytes both by their phenotype and their expression profile [36]. Hemangioma pericytes have increased proliferation, increased vessel formation in vivo, and decreased ability to suppress proliferation and migration of endothelial cells. In addition, the cells secrete more VEGF-A, a critical cytokine for IH proliferation [36, 37].

Propranolol Treatment

Historically, systemic glucocorticoids were the mainstay therapy for complicated IH, with interferon alfa and vincristine used for unresponsive tumors. However, in recent years, beta-blockers, most specifically propranolol, have become the first line treatment. In 2008, Leaute-Labreze et al. published their serendipitous discovery of the rapid clinical effect of propranolol on IHs. In two children treated with propranolol for cardiopulmonary indications [38] rapid regression of the tumor was observed. Since then, many retrospective studies and case reports [39, 40] and few, placebo-controlled trials [41, 42] have supported the efficacy of this treatment. A meta-analysis of 35 studies comprising 795 patients treated with propranolol showed response rate of 97%, compared to pooled response rate of 69% to steroids after 12 months of follow-up ($p < 0.001$) [43]. The dosing is most frequently 2 mg/kg of body weight per day and there is still a lack of consensus regarding the protocols for initiation of the drug and ongoing monitoring [44, 45]. Propranolol use is not devoid of side effects. These include diarrhea, sleep disorders, bronchial hyperreactivity, cold hands and feet as well as—rarely—hypoglycemia that may be life threatening [41, 46]. Consequently, a number of beta blockers other than propranolol (e.g. timolol and nadolol and atenolol) showed similar efficacy with potentially fewer adverse side-effects [47, 48].

Beta Adrenergic Signaling

The β-adrenergic signaling pathway mediates fight-or-flight stress responses through the sympathetic nervous system (SNS) [49]. The sympathetic nerve fibers innervate all tissues in the body and secrete the catecholamine neurotransmitter norepinephrine (NE) in response to environmental , psychological or physiological stimuli [50, 51]. Upon activation, catecholamine levels rises both in tissues and in circulating blood via the release of epinephrine (E) from the adrenal medulla chromaffin cells and NE overflow from vascular neuro-muscular junctions.

The biological effects of NE and E are mediated by three receptor families: $\alpha 1$, $\alpha 2$ and β -adrenergic receptors. Ligation of β-receptors by NE and E activates the $G\alpha s$ guanine nucleotide-binding protein to stimulate adenylyl cyclase synthesis of cyclic $3'-5'$ adenosine monophosphate (cAMP). Subsequently, protein kinase A (PKA) is activated and, in turn, phosphorylates serine or threonine residues on myriad of target proteins involved in cells proliferation, differentiation, morphology and motility. Gene expression studies have demonstrated that approximately 20% of human genes are affected by PKA-induced phosphorylation [52, 53]. An additional key effector of cAMP is guanine nucleotide Exchange Protein activated by Adenylyl Cyclase (EPAC). EPAC stimulates the Ras-like guanine triphosphatase Rap1A, which then activates downstream effectors B-Raf, MEK1/2, and ERK1/2A [54]. Propranolol is an orthosteric antagonist of both $\beta 1$- and $\beta 2$-adrenergic receptors. In addition, it functions as central serotonin 5-HT receptor antagonist, inhibitor of noradrenaline reuptake and indirect agonist of α-adrenergic receptors [55]. The drug exists as a pair of optical isomers: S($-$)propranolol and R($+$)propranolol. The enantiomers bind with relatively large differences in affinity to the β-adrenoceptors [55]. Propranolol, as other pharmacological antagonists of the adrenergic receptors, counteract the agonists via the same signaling pathways.

Stress and the β-adrenergic system have been shown to have many effects on tumor biology. Though with some conflicting results, the use of β-blockers has been linked to increased survival of patients with solid cancers [56]. In addition, stressful life conditions have been shown to correlate with less favorable prognosis of cancer patients. In mouse models of tumors β-adrenergic agonists have also been found accelerate tumor progression and metastasis [57, 58]. As expected by the high percentage of cAMP responsive genes, many cellular processes in tumors were shown to be modulated by the β-adrenergic system, including expression of pro-inflammatory cytokines, of macrophages recruitment, angiogenesis, invasiveness and apoptosis [51, 59].

The study of the mechanism of action of propranolol on IH is much "Younger". Yet, much progress has achieved during recent years. Studies done on human cells isolated from IH in vitro and in vivo, on mouse models, revealed an effect on three major processes that will be detailed below: vascular tone, angiogenesis and vascuogenesis.

Vascular Tone

Following the administration of propranolol, a rapid change in the tumor consistency and color is typically noticed, especially with deep-seated IH [40, 60]. This raises the question of whether propranolol has an effect on the tumor vacular tone via vasoconstriction. Indeed, propranolol has been shown to decrease tissue blood flow to many organs following single administration [61–63]. Particularly in the skin, adrenaline-induced vasoconstriction has been shown to be increased by oral propranolol [64]. However, additional mechanisms might be involved in the slower, long-term effect of propranolol. A potential target of this mechanism of action is the pericyte. Pericytes are regulators of microvascular tone. Bosclo et al. demonstrated that pericytes from proliferating IH have lower density of the cytoskeleton component F-actin fiber compared to involuting Hemangioma pericytes and retinal pericytes. Also, these cells exhibit lower contractile capacity compared to normal pericytes [36]. In another work from the same group Lee et al. demonstrated that Epinephrine-induced relaxation of IH pericytes was prevented by propranolol. Using siRNA assay it was demonstrated that both the relaxation and its prevention by propranolol were mediated by the β2 receptor [65]. Interestingly, cultured pericytes from other sources have been shown to constrict, not relax, in response to catecholamines [66, 67]. Thus, the response of pericytes to NE and its blockers might be cell and context dependent.

In addition to direct effect of propranolol on the pericytes to induce contraction, it might exert its effect indirectly via the blocking of Nitric oxide release from HemEC. The endothelial isoform of nitric-oxide synthase (eNOS), is a key determinant of vascular tone. [68, 69] In different tissues and experimental systems, diverse adrenergic receptors subtypes have been shown to modulate of eNOS expression and activity, including the β1, 2 and 3 adrenergic receptors [70, 71], eNOS protein expression has been demonstrated to be significantly decreased in involuting versus proliferating hemangiomas [72]. In patients treated with propranolol, a significant decrease in the expression of eNOS in hemangioma tissues was noted compared with the age-matched untreated controls [72]. In addition, Wei-li Yuan have shown that serum concentrations of eNOS declined gradually during the first 2 months of propranolol treatment for IH [73].

Angiogenesis

Vascular endothelial growth factor (VEGF) has been shown to play a pivotal role in the angiogenic process in general and specifically in IH proliferation. The VEGF family consists of five ligands VEGF-A, VEGF-B, VEGF-C, VEGF-D and placental growth factor (PIGF). These ligands bind to three main subtypes of VEGF receptors: VEGFR-1 (Flt-1), VEGFR-2 (KDR/Flk-1)and VEGFR-3 [74]. Several works showed over-expression of VEGF-A in proliferating hemangioma tissue and in serum of patients with IH, compared to healthy controls [37, 75–77]. Moreover, we have shown that silencing the expression of VEGF-A in HemSC by short hairpin RNA (shRNA) was sufficient to block blood vessel formation in vivo [37]. NE enhances VEGF-A expression of both normal and tumoral cell types, [78–80]. Propranolol has been shown to reverse this effect via the blocking β1 and β2 adrenergic receptors [78–81]. Several lines of evidence suggest that propranolol acts at least in part through the blocking of VEGF. First, serum VEGF levels were shown to decrease noticeably in 91% of patients after a single month of propranolol treatment [82]. Similar results were reported by another group following the administration of relatively low doses of propranolol [73]. Second, in vitro studies have demonstrated that the NE agonist isoprenaline increased the expression of VEGF-A and the phosphorylation of VEGFR-2 in HemECs in a β-adrenergic receptor- and extracellular-signal-regulated kinase (ERK) -dependent manner. This response was blocked by β-adrenergic blockers. In HemSC, Ling Zhang et al. showed that propranolol at physiological concentrations leads to dose-dependent suppression of VEGF expression, at the mRNA and the protein level [83].

An additional major regulator of angiogenesis is Hypoxia-inducible factor (HIF)-1α. During hypoxia, HIF-1α binds the regulatory region of the VEGF gene, inducing its transcription and initiating its expression [84, 85]. HIF-1α expression has shown to be increased in the endothelium of proliferating hemangioma compared with involuting tissues [77]. Recently, it has been shown that HIF-1α was upregulated in the serum, urine and tumor tissues of IH, and treatment of propranolol markedly inhibited its expression. In vitro, in HemEC, overexpression of HIF-1α blocked the inhibitory effects of propranolol on VEGF expression [86].

Several groups have demonstrated a direct pro-apoptotic or anti proliferative effect of propranolol on HemEC. However, a major concern is the high concentrations of propranolol required for these effects. These drug levels are unlikely to be present in the tumor's microenvironment [87]. It is possible, though, that propranolol works by opposing the growth promoting effects of catecholamines. Ji et al. showed that HemECs proliferation increased in response to isoprenaline via regulation of thee cell-cycle proteins cyclin D1 and its associated kinases, CDK-4 and CDK-6. These effects were reversed by β-adrenergic receptor antagonists. Of note, the antagonists had no effect on basal cell proliferation, but significantly decreased ISO-induced cell proliferation and cell viability [88]

Vasculogenesis

Vasculogenesis, the creation of blood vessels de-novo from stem/progenitor cells, contributes the proliferation of IH. Thus, it is appealing to hypothesize that propranolol acts as an inhibitor of this process, as was shown for corticosteroids and rapamycin [89]. Against this hypothesis is the fact that late regrowth of the hemangioma seen in a subset of patients after cessation of the treatment [90]. This might mean that propranolol does not target the HemSC or even prevents their terminal differentiation or apoptosis. Effect of the adrenergic system on non-hemangioma stem/mesenchymal cells has been shown by several works. For example, NE has been shown to induce brown adipocyte differentiation of mesenchymal progenitors within white adipose tissue [91]. Also, an effect of NE on mesenchymal stem cells adipogenesis has been demonstrated in-vitro cell [92]. In work done on HemSC, Wong et al. reported that Propranolol-treated cells had a more robust response to adipogenic induction when compared to vehicle-treated HemSCs [93]. In a follow-up work the same group has shown that this adipogenic differentiation is characterized by improper adipogenic gene expression [94]. Similar results were reported by another group [95]. However, these results were achieved in very high, non-physiological concentration of propranolol.

Concluding Remarks

Although benign, IH commonly leads to disfigurement and negatively affects the life quality of patients and their families. The discovery of beta blockers have revolutionized the field and offered effective treatment for these lesions. However, not all tumors respond and their use is not without risk. Understanding the pathogenesis of IH and the mechanisms of action of beta blockers could potentially lead to novel pharmacological approaches which are safer and more effective. Advances have been made in recent years, mainly through the isolation and characterization of the cellular components of IH and the creation of relevant animal models. However, due to the complexity of the adrenergic system, more studies are needed in order to establish the relevance of each signaling pathway and cellular effect.

References

1. Haggstrom AN, Drolet BA, Baselga E, Chamlin SL, Garzon MC, Horii KA, Lucky AW, Mancini AJ, Metry DW, Newell B, et al. Prospective study of infantile hemangiomas: demographic, prenatal, and perinatal characteristics. J Pediatr. 2007;150(3):291–4.
2. Amir J, Metzker A, Krikler R, Reisner SH. Strawberry hemangioma in preterm infants. Pediatr Dermatol. 1986;3(4):331–2.
3. Enjolras O, Mulliken JB. The current management of vascular birthmarks. Pediatr Dermatol. 1993;10(4):311–3.
4. Frieden IJ, Haggstrom AN, Drolet BA, Mancini AJ, Friedlander SF, Boon L, Chamlin SL, Baselga E, Garzon MC, Nopper AJ, et al. Infantile hemangiomas: current knowledge, future directions. Proceedings of a research workshop on infantile hemangiomas, April 7-9, 2005, Bethesda, Maryland, USA. Pediatric dermatology. 2005;22(5):383–406.
5. Chang LC, Haggstrom AN, Drolet BA, Baselga E, Chamlin SL, Garzon MC, Horii KA, Lucky AW, Mancini AJ, Metry DW, et al. Growth characteristics of infantile hemangiomas: implications for management. Pediatrics. 2008;122(2):360–7.
6. Bruckner AL, Frieden IJ. Hemangiomas of infancy. J Am Acad Dermatol. 2003;48(4):477–93; quiz 494–6.
7. Drolet BA, Esterly NB, Frieden IJ. Hemangiomas in children. N Engl J Med. 1999;341(3):173–81.
8. Dosanjh A, Chang J, Bresnick S, Zhou L, Reinisch J, Longaker M, Karasek M. In vitro characteristics of neonatal hemangioma endothelial cells: similarities and differences between normal neonatal and fetal endothelial cells. J Cutan Pathol. 2000;27(9):441–50.
9. Razon MJ, Kraling BM, Mulliken JB, Bischoff J. Increased apoptosis coincides with onset of involution in infantile hemangioma. Microcirculation. 1998;5(2-3):189–95.
10. Iwata J, Sonobe H, Furihata M, Ido E, Ohtsuki Y. High frequency of apoptosis in infantile capillary haemangioma. J Pathol. 1996;179(4):403–8.
11. North PE, Waner M, Mizeracki A, Mrak RE, Nicholas R, Kincannon J, Suen JY, Mihm Jr MC. A unique microvascular phenotype shared by juvenile hemangiomas and human placenta. Arch Dermatol. 2001;137(5):559–70.
12. Barnes CM, Huang S, Kaipainen A, Sanoudou D, Chen EJ, Eichler GS, Guo Y, Yu Y, Ingber DE, Mulliken JB, et al. Evidence by molecular profiling for a placental origin of infantile hemangioma. Proc Natl Acad Sci U S A. 2005;102(52):19097–102.
13. Huang SA, Tu HM, Harney JW, Venihaki M, Butte AJ, Kozakewich HP, Fishman SJ, Larsen PR. Severe hypothyroidism caused by type 3 iodothyronine deiodinase in infantile hemangiomas. N Engl J Med. 2000;343(3):185–9.

14. Alfirevic Z, Sundberg K, Brigham S. Amniocentesis and chorionic villus sampling for prenatal diagnosis. Cochrane Database Syst Rev. 2003(3):CD003252.
15. Bauland CG, Smit JM, Bartelink LR, Zondervan HA, Spauwen PH. Hemangioma in the newborn: increased incidence after chorionic villus sampling. Prenat Diagn. 2010;30(10):913–7.
16. Khan ZA, Boscolo E, Picard A, Psutka S, Melero-Martin JM, Bartch TC, Mulliken JB, Bischoff J. Multipotential stem cells recapitulate human infantile hemangioma in immunodeficient mice. J Clin Invest. 2008;118(7):2592–9.
17. Boscolo E, Stewart CL, Greenberger S, Wu JK, Durham JT, Herman IM, Mulliken JB, Kitajewski J, Bischoff J. JAGGED1 signaling regulates hemangioma stem cell-to-pericyte/vascular smooth muscle cell differentiation. Arterioscler Thromb Vasc Biol. 2011;31(10): 2181–92.
18. Xu D, TM O, Shartava A, Fowles TC, Yang J, Fink LM, Ward DC, Mihm MC, Waner M, Ma Y. Isolation, characterization, and in vitro propagation of infantile hemangioma stem cells and an in vivo mouse model. J Hematol Oncol. 2011;4:54.
19. Itinteang T, Brasch HD, Tan ST, Day DJ. Expression of components of the renin-angiotensin system in proliferating infantile haemangioma may account for the propranolol-induced accelerated involution. J Plastic Recons Aesthetic Surg JPRAS. 2011;64(6):759–65.
20. Spock CL, Tom LK, Canadas K, Sue GR, Sawh-Martinez R, Maier CL, Pober JS, Galan A, Schultz B, Waner M, et al. Infantile hemangiomas exhibit neural crest and pericyte markers. Ann Plast Surg. 2015;74(2):230–6.
21. Hopel-Kreiner I. Histogenesis of hemangiomas – an ultrastructural study on capillary and cavernous hemangiomas of the skin. Pathol Res Pract. 1980;170:70.
22. Boye E, Yu Y, Paranya G, Mulliken JB, Olsen BR, Bischoff J. Clonality and altered behavior of endothelial cells from hemangiomas. J Clin Invest. 2001;107(6):745–52.
23. Greenberger S, Bischoff J. Pathogenesis of infantile haemangioma. Br J Dermatol. 2013;169(1):12–9.
24. North PE, Waner M, Mizeracki A, Mihm Jr MC. GLUT1: a newly discovered immunohistochemical marker for juvenile hemangiomas. Hum Pathol. 2000;31(1):11–22.
25. Yu Y, Varughese J, Brown LF, Mulliken JB, Bischoff J. Increased Tie2 expression, enhanced response to angiopoietin-1, and dysregulated angiopoietin-2 expression in hemangioma-derived endothelial cells. Am J Pathol. 2001;159(6):2271–80.
26. Yu Y, Flint AF, Mulliken JB, Wu JK, Bischoff J. Endothelial progenitor cells in infantile hemangioma. Blood. 2004;103(4):1373–5.
27. Wang FQ, Chen G, Zhu JY, Zhang W, Ren JG, Liu H, Sun ZJ, Jia J, Zhao YF. M2-polarised macrophages in infantile haemangiomas: correlation with promoted angiogenesis. J Clin Pathol. 2013;66(12):1058–64.
28. Ritter MR, Reinisch J, Friedlander SF, Friedlander M. Myeloid cells in infantile hemangioma. Am J Pathol. 2006;168(2):621–8.
29. Mills CD. M1 and M2 Macrophages: oracles of health and disease. Crit Rev Immunol. 2012;32(6):463–88.
30. Zhang W, Chen G, Wang FQ, Ren JG, Zhu JY, Cai Y, Zhao JH, Jia J, Zhao YF. Macrophages contribute to the progression of infantile hemangioma by regulating the proliferation and differentiation of hemangioma stem cells. J Invest Dermatol. 2015;135(12):3163–72.
31. Crisan M, Yap S, Casteilla L, Chen CW, Corselli M, Park TS, Andriolo G, Sun B, Zheng B, Zhang L, et al. A perivascular origin for mesenchymal stem cells in multiple human organs. Cell Stem Cell. 2008;3(3):301–13.
32. Crisan M, Corselli M, Chen WC, Peault B. Perivascular cells for regenerative medicine. J Cell Mol Med. 2012;16(12):2851–60.
33. Ribatti D, Nico B, Crivellato E. The role of pericytes in angiogenesis. Inter J Devel Biol. 2011;55(3):261–8.
34. van Dijk CG, Nieuweboer FE, Pei JY, Xu YJ, Burgisser P, van Mulligen E, el Azzouzi H, Duncker DJ, Verhaar MC, Cheng C. The complex mural cell: pericyte function in health and disease. Int J Cardiol. 2015;190:75–89.

35. Kutcher ME, Herman IM. The pericyte: cellular regulator of microvascular blood flow. Microvasc Res. 2009;77(3):235–46.
36. Boscolo E, Mulliken JB, Bischoff J. Pericytes from infantile hemangioma display proangiogenic properties and dysregulated angiopoietin-1. Arterioscler Thromb Vasc Biol. 2013;33(3):501–9.
37. Greenberger S, Boscolo E, Adini I, Mulliken JB, Bischoff J. Corticosteroid suppression of VEGF-A in infantile hemangioma-derived stem cells. N Engl J Med. 2010;362(11):1005–13. doi: 10.1056/NEJMoa0903036. PMID: 20237346. Free PMC Article.
38. Leaute-Labreze C, Dumas de la Roque E, Hubiche T, Boralevi F, Thambo JB, Taieb A. Propranolol for severe hemangiomas of infancy. N Engl J Med. 2008;358(24):2649–51.
39. Price CJ, Lattouf C, Baum B, McLeod M, Schachner LA, Duarte AM, Connelly EA. Propranolol vs corticosteroids for infantile hemangiomas: a multicenter retrospective analysis. Arch Dermatol. 2011;147(12):1371–6.
40. Sans V, de la Roque ED, Berge J, Grenier N, Boralevi F, Mazereeuw-Hautier J, Lipsker D, Dupuis E, Ezzedine K, Vergnes P, et al. Propranolol for severe infantile hemangiomas: follow-up report. Pediatrics. 2009;124(3):e423–31.
41. Leaute-Labreze C, Hoeger P, Mazereeuw-Hautier J, Guibaud L, Baselga E, Posiunas G, Phillips RJ, Caceres H, Lopez Gutierrez JC, Ballona R, et al. A randomized, controlled trial of oral propranolol in infantile hemangioma. N Engl J Med. 2015;372(8):735–46.
42. Hogeling M, Adams S, Wargon O. A randomized controlled trial of propranolol for infantile hemangiomas. Pediatrics. 2011;128(2):e259–66.
43. Izadpanah A, Kanevsky J, Belzile E, Schwarz K. Propranolol versus corticosteroids in the treatment of infantile hemangioma: a systematic review and meta-analysis. Plast Reconstr Surg. 2013;131(3):601–13.
44. Biesbroeck L, Brandling-Bennett HA. Propranolol for infantile haemangiomas: review of report of a consensus conference. Arch Dis Child Educ Pract Ed. 2014;99(3):95–7.
45. Drolet BA, Frommelt PC, Chamlin SL, Haggstrom A, Bauman NM, Chiu YE, Chun RH, Garzon MC, Holland KE, Liberman L, et al. Initiation and use of propranolol for infantile hemangioma: report of a consensus conference. Pediatrics. 2013;131(1):128–40.
46. Horev A, Haim A, Zvulunov A. Propranolol induced hypoglycemia. Pediatr Endocrinol Rev. 2015;12(3):308-10.
47. Abarzua-Araya A, Navarrete-Dechent CP, Heusser F, Retamal J, Zegpi-Trueba MS. Atenolol versus propranolol for the treatment of infantile hemangiomas: a randomized controlled study. J Am Acad Dermatol. 2014;70(6):1045–9.
48. Pope E, Chakkittakandiyil A, Lara-Corrales I, Maki E, Weinstein M. Expanding the therapeutic repertoire of infantile haemangiomas: cohort-blinded study of oral nadolol compared with propranolol. Br J Dermatol. 2013;168(1):222–4.
49. Madamanchi A. Beta-adrenergic receptor signaling in cardiac function and heart failure. McGill J Med MJM Inter Forum Adv Med Sci Students. 2007;10(2):99–104.
50. Daly CJ, McGrath JC. Previously unsuspected widespread cellular and tissue distribution of beta-adrenoceptors and its relevance to drug action. Trends Pharmacol Sci. 2011;32(4):219–26.
51. Cole SW, Sood AK. Molecular pathways: beta-adrenergic signaling in cancer. Clin Cancer Res. 2012;18(5):1201–6.
52. Montminy M. Transcriptional regulation by cyclic AMP. Annu Rev Biochem. 1997;66:807–22.
53. Zhang X, Odom DT, Koo SH, Conkright MD, Canettieri G, Best J, Chen H, Jenner R, Herbolsheimer E, Jacobsen E, et al. Genome-wide analysis of cAMP-response element binding protein occupancy, phosphorylation, and target gene activation in human tissues. Proc Natl Acad Sci U S A. 2005;102(12):4459–64.
54. de Rooij J, Zwartkruis FJ, Verheijen MH, Cool RH, Nijman SM, Wittinghofer A, Bos JL. Epac is a Rap1 guanine-nucleotide-exchange factor directly activated by cyclic AMP. Nature. 1998;396(6710):474–7.

55. Young R, Glennon RA. S(−)Propranolol as a discriminative stimulus and its comparison to the stimulus effects of cocaine in rats. Psychopharmacol. 2009;203(2):369–82.
56. Watkins JL, Thaker PH, Nick AM, Ramondetta LM, Kumar S, Urbauer DL, Matsuo K, Squires KC, Coleman RL, Lutgendorf SK, et al. Clinical impact of selective and nonselective beta-blockers on survival in patients with ovarian cancer. Cancer. 2015;121(19):3444–51.
57. Sloan EK, Priceman SJ, Cox BF, Yu S, Pimentel MA, Tangkanangnukul V, Arevalo JM, Morizono K, Karanikolas BD, Wu L, et al. The sympathetic nervous system induces a meta-static switch in primary breast cancer. Cancer Res. 2010;70(18):7042–52.
58. Thaker PH, Han LY, Kamat AA, Arevalo JM, Takahashi R, Lu C, Jennings NB, Armaiz-Pena G, Bankson JA, Ravoori M, et al. Chronic stress promotes tumor growth and angiogenesis in a mouse model of ovarian carcinoma. Nat Med. 2006;12(8):939–44.
59. Tang J, Li Z, Lu L, Cho CH. beta-Adrenergic system, a backstage manipulator regulating tumour progression and drug target in cancer therapy. Semin Cancer Biol. 2013;23(6 Pt B):533–42.
60. Rosbe KW, Suh KY, Meyer AK, Maguiness SM, Frieden IJ. Propranolol in the management of airway infantile hemangiomas. Arch Otolaryngol Head Neck Surg. 2010;136(7):658–65.
61. Nies AS, Evans GH, Shand DG. Regional hemodynamic effects of beta-adrenergic blockade with propranolol in the unanesthetized primate. Am Heart J. 1973;85(1):97–102.
62. McSorley PD, Warren DJ. Effects of propranolol and metoprolol on the peripheral circulation. Br Med J. 1978;2(6152):1598–600.
63. Vandenburg MJ, Conlon C, Ledingham JM. A comparison of the effects of propranolol and oxprenolol on forearm blood flow and skin temperature. Br J Clin Pharmacol. 1981;11(5):485–90.
64. Doshi BS, Kulkarni RD, Dattani KK, Anand MP. Effect of labetalol and propranolol on human cutaneous vasoconstrictor response to adrenaline. Int J Clin Pharmacol Res. 1984;4(1):25–8.
65. Lee D, Boscolo E, Durham JT, Mulliken JB, Herman IM, Bischoff J. Propranolol targets the contractility of infantile haemangioma-derived pericytes. Br J Dermatol. 2014;171(5):1129–37.
66. Kelley C, D'Amore P, Hechtman HB, Shepro D. Vasoactive hormones and cAMP affect pericyte contraction and stress fibres in vitro. J Muscle Res Cell Motil. 1988;9(2):184–94.
67. Markhotina N, Liu GJ, Martin DK. Contractility of retinal pericytes grown on silicone elastomer substrates is through a protein kinase A-mediated intracellular pathway in response to vasoactive peptides. IET Nanobiotechnol IET. 2007;1(3):44–51.
68. Balligand JL, Cannon PJ. Nitric oxide synthases and cardiac muscle. Autocrine and paracrine influences. Arterioscler Thromb Vasc Biol. 1997;17(10):1846–58.
69. McHugh J, Cheek DJ. Nitric oxide and regulation of vascular tone: pharmacological and physiological considerations. Am J Crit Care Off Pub Am Asso Crit Care Nurses. 1998;7(2):131–40; quiz 141–2.
70. Ferro A, Coash M, Yamamoto T, Rob J, Ji Y, Queen L. Nitric oxide-dependent beta2-adrenergic dilatation of rat aorta is mediated through activation of both protein kinase A and Akt. Br J Pharmacol. 2004;143(3):397–403.
71. Dessy C, Saliez J, Ghisdal P, Daneau G, Lobysheva II, Frerart F, Belge C, Jnaoui K, Noirhomme P, Feron O, et al. Endothelial beta3-adrenoreceptors mediate nitric oxide-dependent vasorelaxation of coronary microvessels in response to the third-generation beta-blocker nebivolol. Circulation. 2005;112(8):1198–205.
72. Dai Y, Hou F, Buckmiller L, Fan CY, Saad A, Suen J, Richter GT. Decreased eNOS protein expression in involuting and propranolol-treated hemangiomas. Arch Otolaryngol Head Neck Surg. 2012;138(2):177–82.
73. Yuan WL, Jin ZL, Wei JJ, Liu ZY, Xue L, Wang XK. Propranolol given orally for proliferating infantile haemangiomas: analysis of efficacy and serological changes in vascular endothelial growth factor and endothelial nitric oxide synthase in 35 patients. Br J Oral Maxillofac Surg. 2013;51(7):656–61.

74. McMahon G. VEGF receptor signaling in tumor angiogenesis. Oncologist. 2000;5(Suppl 1):3–10.
75. Takahashi K, Mulliken JB, Kozakewich HP, Rogers RA, Folkman J, Ezekowitz RA. Cellular markers that distinguish the phases of hemangioma during infancy and childhood. J Clin Invest. 1994;93(6):2357–64.
76. Chang J, Most D, Bresnick S, Mehrara B, Steinbrech DS, Reinisch J, Longaker MT, Turk AE. Proliferative hemangiomas: analysis of cytokine gene expression and angiogenesis. Plast Reconstr Surg. 1999;103(1):1–9; discussion 10.
77. Kleinman ME, Greives MR, Churgin SS, Blechman KM, Chang EI, Ceradini DJ, Tepper OM, Gurtner GC. Hypoxia-induced mediators of stem/progenitor cell trafficking are increased in children with hemangioma. Arterioscler Thromb Vasc Biol. 2007;27(12):2664–70.
78. Fredriksson JM, Lindquist JM, Bronnikov GE, Nedergaard J. Norepinephrine induces vascular endothelial growth factor gene expression in brown adipocytes through a beta -adrenoreceptor/cAMP/protein kinase a pathway involving Src but independently of Erk1/2. J Biol Chem. 2000;275(18):13802–11.
79. Lutgendorf SK, Cole S, Costanzo E, Bradley S, Coffin J, Jabbari S, Rainwater K, Ritchie JM, Yang M, Sood AK. Stress-related mediators stimulate vascular endothelial growth factor secretion by two ovarian cancer cell lines. Clin Cancer Res. 2003;9(12):4514–21.
80. Park SY, Kang JH, Jeong KJ, Lee J, Han JW, Choi WS, Kim YK, Kang J, Park CG, Lee HY. Norepinephrine induces VEGF expression and angiogenesis by a hypoxia-inducible factor-1alpha protein-dependent mechanism. Int J Cancer. 2011;128(10):2306–16.
81. Guo K, Ma Q, Wang L, Hu H, Li J, Zhang D, Zhang M. Norepinephrine-induced invasion by pancreatic cancer cells is inhibited by propranolol. Oncol Rep. 2009;22(4):825–30.
82. Chen XD, Ma G, Huang JL, Chen H, Jin YB, Ye XX, Hu XJ, Lin XX. Serum-level changes of vascular endothelial growth factor in children with infantile hemangioma after oral propranolol therapy. Pediatr Dermatol. 2013;30(5):549–53.
83. Zhang L, Mai HM, Zheng J, Zheng JW, Wang YA, Qin ZP, Li KL. Propranolol inhibits angiogenesis via down-regulating the expression of vascular endothelial growth factor in hemangioma derived stem cell. Inter J Clin Exp Pathol. 2014;7(1):48–55.
84. Ziello JE, Jovin IS, Huang Y. Hypoxia-Inducible Factor (HIF)-1 regulatory pathway and its potential for therapeutic intervention in malignancy and ischemia. Yale J Biol Med. 2007;80(2):51–60.
85. Dery MA, Michaud MD, Richard DE. Hypoxia-inducible factor 1: regulation by hypoxic and non-hypoxic activators. Int J Biochem Cell Biol. 2005;37(3):535–40.
86. Li P, Guo Z, Gao Y, Pan W. Propranolol represses infantile hemangioma cell growth through the beta2-adrenergic receptor in a HIF-1alpha-dependent manner. Oncol Rep. 2015;33(6):3099–107.
87. Wong L, Nation RL, Chiou WL, Mehta PK. Plasma concentrations of propranolol and 4-hydroxypropranolol during chronic oral propranolol therapy. Br J Clin Pharmacol. 1979;8(2):163–7.
88. Ji Y, Chen S, Li K, Xiao X, Zheng S, Xu T. The role of beta-adrenergic receptor signaling in the proliferation of hemangioma-derived endothelial cells. Cell Div. 2013;8(1):1.
89. Greenberger S, Yuan S, Walsh LA, Boscolo E, Kang KT, Matthews B, Mulliken JB, Bischoff J. Rapamycin suppresses self-renewal and vasculogenic potential of stem cells isolated from infantile hemangioma. J Invest Dermatol. 2011;131(12):2467–76.
90. Bagazgoitia L, Hernandez-Martin A, Torrelo A. Recurrence of infantile hemangiomas treated with propranolol. Pediatr Dermatol. 2011;28(6):658–62.
91. Vegiopoulos A, Muller-Decker K, Strzoda D, Schmitt I, Chichelnitskiy E, Ostertag A, Berriel Diaz M, Rozman J, Hrabe de Angelis M, Nusing RM, et al. Cyclooxygenase-2 controls energy homeostasis in mice by de novo recruitment of brown adipocytes. Science New York NY. 2010;328(5982):1158–61.

92. Li H, Fong C, Chen Y, Cai G, Yang M. beta2- and beta3-, but not beta1-adrenergic receptors are involved in osteogenesis of mouse mesenchymal stem cells via cAMP/PKA signaling. Arch Biochem Biophys. 2010;496(2):77–83.
93. Wong A, Hardy KL, Kitajewski AM, Shawber CJ, Kitajewski JK, Wu JK. Propranolol accelerates adipogenesis in hemangioma stem cells and causes apoptosis of hemangioma endothelial cells. Plast Reconstr Surg. 2012;130(5):1012–21.
94. England RW, Hardy KL, Kitajewski AM, Wong A, Kitajewski JK, Shawber CJ, Wu JK. Propranolol promotes accelerated and dysregulated adipogenesis in hemangioma stem cells. Ann Plast Surg. 2014;73(Suppl 1):S119–24.
95. Ma X, Zhao T, Ouyang T, Xin S, Ma Y, Chang M. Propranolol enhanced adipogenesis instead of induction of apoptosis of hemangiomas stem cells. Inter J Clin Exp Pathol. 2014;7(7):3809–17.

The Role of Angiogenesis in the Development of Psoriasis

Ana Carolina Belini Bazan-Arruda, Daniela Melo Siqueira, and Larissa Mondadori Mercadante

Introduction

Psoriasis is an immune-mediated, inflammatory dermatosis. In susceptible patients, both environmental and genetic factors contribute to the symptom development of this chronic, debilitating disease [1, 2]. With many known clinical subtypes, it is characterized by the presence of erythematous plaques, covered by silvery scales. Angiogenesis plays an important role in this disease pathogenesis, with vascular alterations being the initial trigger to the autoimmune inflammatory response [1]. In this chapter, we present the latest work on the main mechanisms through which angiogenesis interfere on the physiopathology of psoriasis.

Historical Aspects

Psoriasis, from the Greek *psora*, pruritus or itch, is a long-known disease [3, 4]. Hippocrates (460–375 b.C.) used the term hypopsorodea in his fourth Epidemics book to describe psoriasis-like lesions, which he named *lopoi* (from *lepo*, desquamate) and classified as squamous eruptions [5, 6].

The first historical report on the disease was given by Celsus (25 b.C.-45 a.C.) [6]. Galen (133–200 a.C.) created the term psoriasis, although his description of eyelid lesions and of other psoriasis-like lesions associated to desquamation and pruritus suggests that this author, in fact, was referring to seborrheic dermatitis [6].

A.C.B. Bazan-Arruda, MD (✉)
Dermatology, Hospital e Maternidade Celso Pierro – PUC-Campinas, Campinas, Brazil
e-mail: acbbazan@yahoo.com.br

D.M. Siqueira, MD • L.M. Mercadante, MD
Dermatology Resident, Hospital e Maternidade Celso Pierro – PUC-Campinas, Campinas, Brazil

© Springer-Verlag London Ltd. 2017
J.L. Arbiser (ed.), *Angiogenesis-Based Dermatology*,
DOI 10.1007/978-1-4471-7314-4_3

Until the end of the eighteenth century, both psoriasis and Hansen's disease were grouped together, with patients suffering the same type of discrimation [6].

In the beginning of the nineteenth century, Robert Willan (1757–1812) described it as a clinical entity, but it was not before four decades later, in 1841, that Ferdinand von Hebra separated Hansen's disease from psoriasis definitely [3, 5, 6].

Finally, it has only been 200 years since the disease has been recognized by a spectrum of clinical variants, which remains barely unchanged [5].

In 1971, while investigating the etiology of psoriasis, Folkman was one of the first to suggest that angiogenesis could contribute to the development of this disease, fact corroborated by several subsequent studies [7].

Epidemiology

Psoriasis affects approximately 125 million people worldwide, representing near 2.2% of the global population [8]. It affects men and women equally and may manifest itself at any age [8, 9]. However, some studies demonstrated that the beginning of symptoms is especially associated to two incidence peaks: age groups 15–20 years and 50-60 years [8, 9]. The prevalence varies depending on the studied population and age group, being higher in countries far from the Equator [8]. Such variability may be explained by genetic susceptibility, climate and exposure to local antigens [10]. It is estimated that psoriasis affects 2–4% of the Occidental population [9]. In the United States of America (USA), near 2% of the population is affected, with a higher prevalence seen on Caucasians when compared to Afro-Americans [8, 9].

Prevalence is low in some ethnic groups, being rare among Japanese and virtually absent in South American Indians and Australian aborigines [8].

Clinical Features

Psoriasis is classified as an erythemato-squamous disease, although clinical manifestations may vary depending on its several subtypes. It is a chronic disorder, characterized by exacerbation and remission periods, from which residual lesions can result [11].

Plaque Psoriasis (Psoriasis Vulgaris)

Found in 90% of patients, it is characterized by well-defined, erythemato-squamous plaques, with dry, silvery-white, adherent scales, showing different degrees of infiltration and size (Figs. 3.1 and 3.2). It mainly affects the extensor surfaces of limbs, the scalp and the sacral region, with occasional pruritus [11].

Nail Psoriasis

The cupuliform depressions called pittings of the nails (thimble nails) are the most observed nail changes and occur due to changes of the proximal nail fold. The

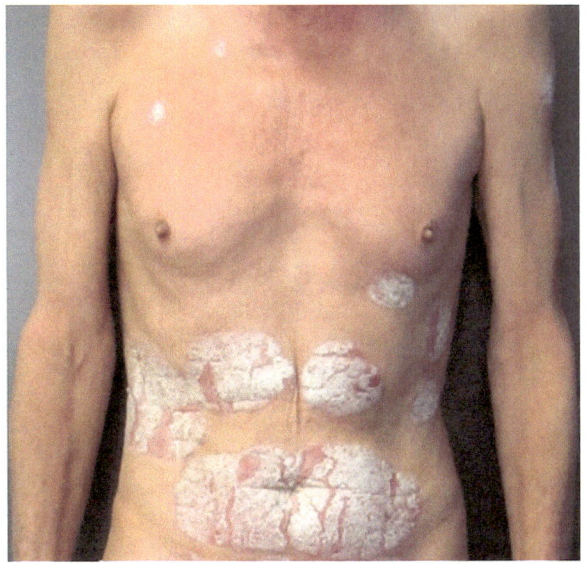

Fig. 3.1 Plaque psoriasis. Archives of the Ambulatório de Psoríase, Pontifícia Universidade Católica de Campinas

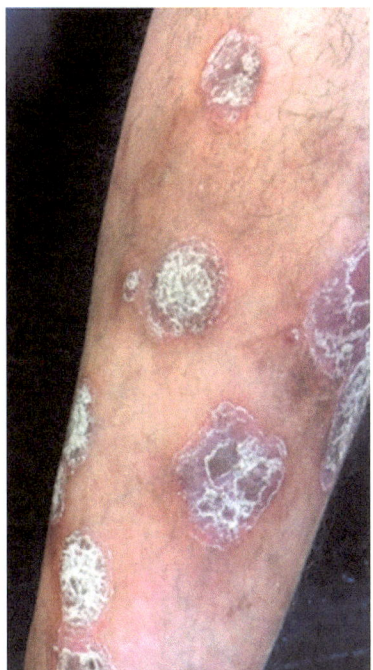

Fig. 3.2 Plaque psoriasis. Archives of the Ambulatório de Psoríase, Pontifícia Universidade Católica de Campinas

involvement of the nail plate can determine the appearance of subungual hyperkeratosis, onycholysis and "oil slicks" (brown band between onycholysis and lunula). The longitudinal ridges and onychodystrophy (Fig. 3.3) are caused by damage to ungueal matrix [11].

Guttate Psoriasis

It is characterized by the sudden appearance of erythemato-squamous papules, usually on the trunk and proximal parts of limbs (Fig. 3.4). Being more common in children, teenagers and young adults, this form of psoriasis may be preceded by streptococcic infections and often heals spontaneously in a few months, although in some cases it may persist and evolve to the plaque form [11].

Erythrodermic Psoriasis

An intense erythema is seen over the entire integument, with variable desquamation (Fig. 3.5). Its occurrence may be due to the natural evolution of the disease in immunosuppressed patients (iatrogenic form) or because of the patient's bad response to

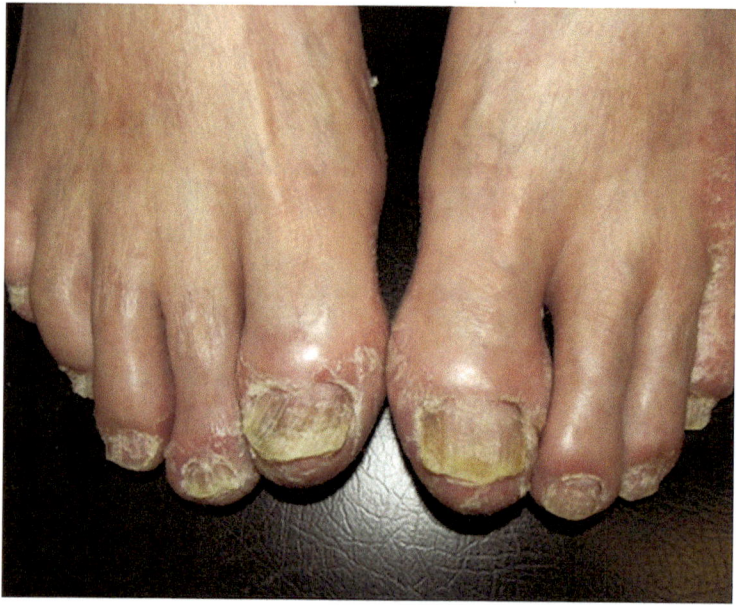

Fig. 3.3 Ungueal psoriasis. Archives of the Ambulatório de Psoríase, Pontifícia Universidade Católica de Campinas

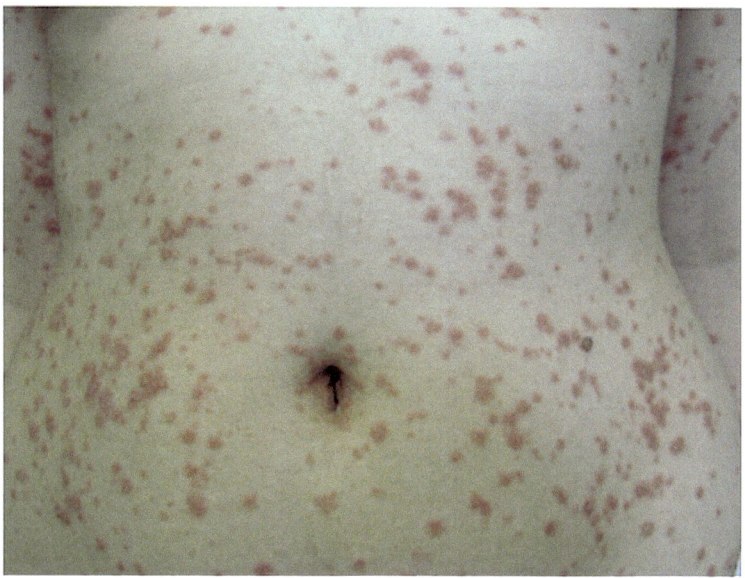

Fig. 3.4 Guttate psoriasis. Archives of the Ambulatório de Psoríase, Pontifícia Universidade Católica de Campinas

treatment. In such a form, it may be systemic and affects the heart, kidneys and liver, in addition to increasing the risk of secondary infections, which requires the patient hospitalization [11].

Pustalar Psoriasis

This form of the disease is characterized by the aggravation of both the erythema and edema of previous lesions, followed by the appearance of confluent, non-follicular, superficial pustules, especially on flexures and the trunk (Fig. 3.6). It may be generalized or localized, and evolves from plaque psoriasis because of treatment interruption, infection or hypokalemia, or assumes an idiopathic form. Its occurrence is acute and patients will relapse within a few weeks [11].

Palmoplantar Psoriasis

This type of psoriasis is more common in adults, being characterized by the appearance of symmetrical, well-defined plaques, showing intense hyperkeratosis. It may form fissures, except on the plantar cavus (Figs. 3.7 and 3.8) [11].

Fig. 3.5 Erythrodermic
psoriasis. Archives of the
Ambulatório de Psoríase,
Pontifícia Universidade
Católica de Campinas

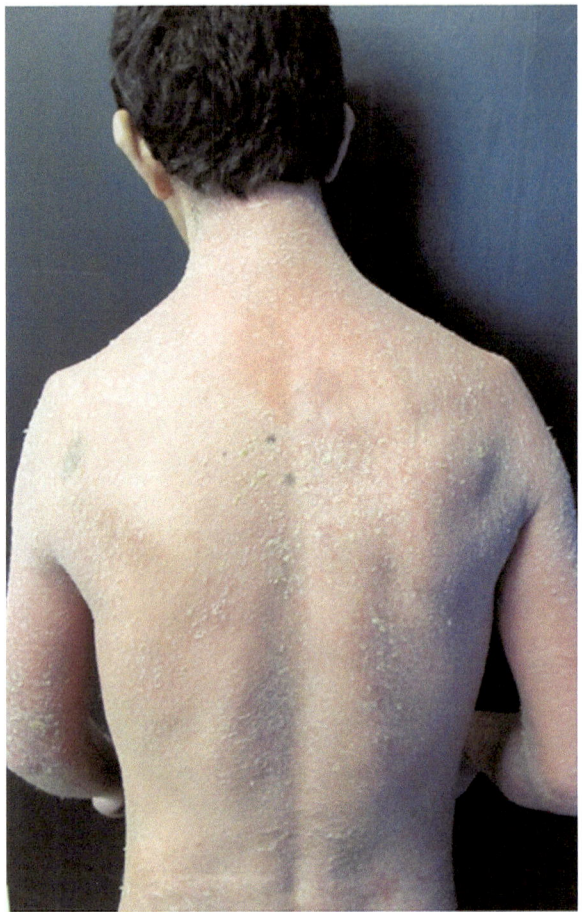

Psoriasis in Children

Atypical presentations may be observed in infants, but it is mostly characterized by a few erythematous plaques with little desquamation, occurring in the perioral, periorbital, the scalp and genital regions (Fig. 3.9). Follicular affection is common. There is no correlation between an early start of the disease and the worst prognosis [11].

Psoriasis in the Elderly

Lesions are mainly observed in inferior limbs and the scalp, with pronounced pruritus. In general, the disorder varies from mild to moderate, but treatment may be impaired by drug interactions [11].

Fig. 3.6 Pustular
psoriasis. Archives of the
Ambulatório de Psoríase,
Pontifícia Universidade
Católica de Campinas

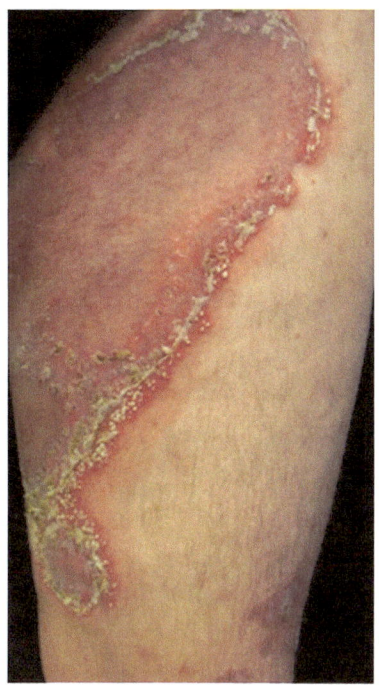

Anatomopathology

In psoriasis, histopathological findings are nonspecific but very characteristic, and may be found in other dermatological diseases, such as in Pityriasis Rubra Pilaris and Lichen Simplex Chronicus [12]. In initial lesions, vascular proliferation and superficial vasodilation are observed in the dermis (Fig. 3.10). The perivascular infiltrate is composed of lymphocytes and macrophages. With plaque development, this infiltrate becomes a mixture of lymphocytes, macrophages and neutrophils, with neutrophils and lymphocytes migrating towards the epidermis. Vascular alterations become even more evident, with an increase in the number and size of capillaries, as well as the acquisition of a tortuous appearance (Fig. 3.11) [13]. In the epidermis, there is an increase in the spinous layer (acanthosis), as seen by the regular elongation of the dermal papillae and epidermal cones (Fig. 3.12). The suprapapillary region becomes thinned and the granular layer may be reduced or absent (hypogranulosis or agranulosis) [12]. In the corneal layer, hyperkeratosis with parakeratosis (because of the increase in nucleated keratinocytes) is evident. Neutrophils that migrated towards the epidermis gather forming Munro's microabscesses in the corneal layer, and spongiform pustules of Kogoj in the spinous layer [12].

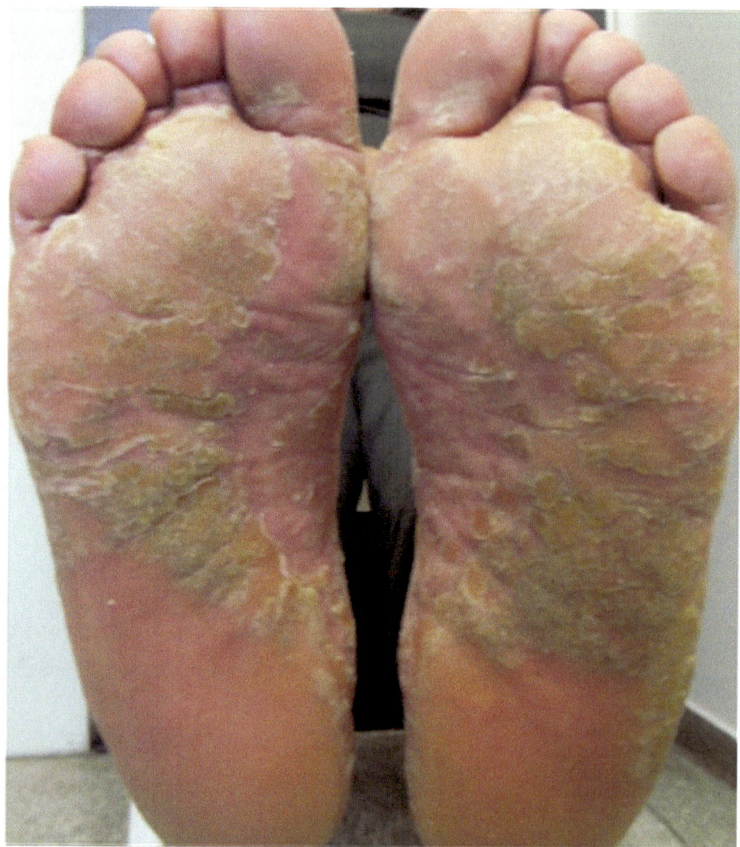

Fig. 3.7 Plantar psoriasis. Archives of the Ambulatório de Psoríase, Pontifícia Universidade Católica de Campinas

Angiogenesis in the Etiopathogenesis of Psoriasis

In spite of the advances in treatment for this chronic, immune-mediated, inflammatory disease, there are still etiological aspects of psoriasis that are not completely understood [14].

Specific cells responsible for triggering psoriasis have not been determined yet, although it is known that T-helper lymphocytes (especially T-helper-1 and T-helper-17) and T regulators contribute to the pro-angiogenic environment fundamental to the beginning and maintenance of the disease [14, 15].

Angiogenesis represents one of the initial events in psoriasis, occurring even before plaque formation [13].

Angiogenesis is the process by which new capillaries form from pre-existing vessels, with the use of the extracellular matrix and the recruitment of pericytes and smooth muscles cells. It occurs physiologically during embryogenesis, the feminine

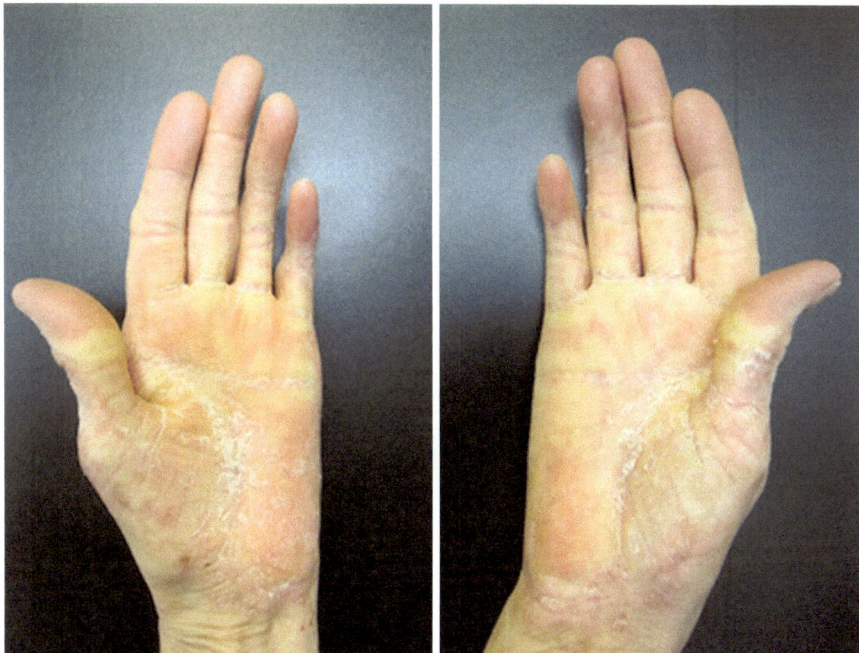

Fig. 3.8 Palmar psoriasis. Archives of the Ambulatório de Psoríase, Pontifícia Universidade Católica de Campinas

menstrual cycle, and in tissue repair and cicatrization processes. Inflammatory diseases, such as psoriasis, and the development of tumors are also marked by angiogenesis.

The papillary dermis of patients with psoriasis presents peculiar histological features, including elongated, tortuous, blood capillaries, increased in diameter and number [16–19]. Such vascular alterations occur prematurely and precede the characteristic epidermal hyperplasia of the disease [17, 20]. Effective treatments normalize this vascular dilation before alterations on the epidermis are seen, but other structural modifications in neo-formed vessels may persist for up to 9 months after clinical improvements are observed [19]. Increases in the cutaneous blood flow caused by angiogenesis are also observed in the clinically healthy skin, surrounding the plaque [21, 22].

Clinically, the dilation and elongation of blood capillaries correspond to the Auspitz's sign. This sign is characterized by the presence of small bleeding points resulting from the mechanical rupture of the neo-formed vessels in the papillary dermis, after the scales have been removed through Brocq's methodic curettage [23].

In addition to the structural alterations of vessels seen in the papillary dermis, there is an increase in the migration of inflammatory cells and in the expression of adherence molecules, such as E-selectin, ICAM-1 (Intercellular Adhesion Molecule 1) and the vascular cell adhesion molecule-1 [24, 25].

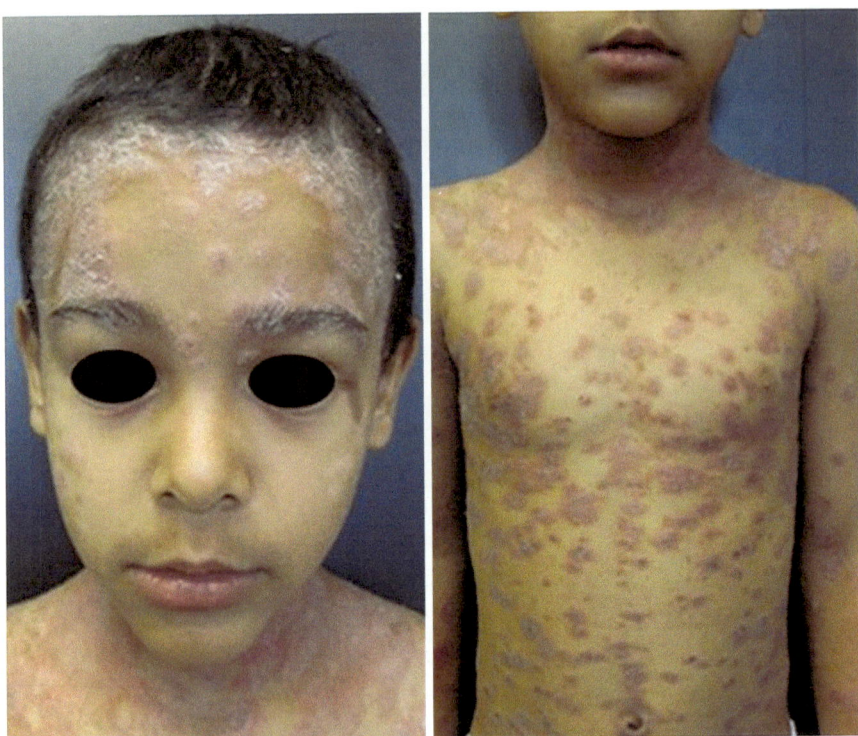

Fig. 3.9 Psoriasis in children. Archives of the Ambulatório de Psoríase, Pontifícia Universidade Católica de Campinas

The strong adhesion of leucocytes to endothelial cells triggers the inflammatory response, coordinated by the infiltrate composed of neutrophils, mastocytes and especially of (CD4+) T-helper lymphocytes, which secrete inflammatory cytokines such as IL-17, tumor necrosis factor (TNF) and gamma interferon (IFN-γ) [7, 26, 27]. In the presence of IFN-γ, the immune response becomes polarized. As a result, a pattern of Th1 and Th17 lymphocytes is formed, an important event in the physiopathology of psoriasis for these cells are responsible for the proliferation of keratinocytes in the epidermis [1, 13].

A study with keratinocytes of both lesioned and non-lesioned skin showed that endothelial cells of sick patients exhibited a greater stimulus to migrate, when compared to those of healthy individuals [28].

During angiogenesis, endothelial cells use the components of the extracellular matrix to migrate [13]. Such a mechanism is mediated by transmembrane, heterodimeric proteins expressed in their walls, the integrins [13]. These proteins are responsible for the activation of intracellular signaling pathways [13] and modulate the pro-angiogenic response [29]. Among integrins, $\alpha_v\beta3$ is expressed in low levels in the normal vascular tree, acting as a receptor for the von Willebrand factor, fibrinogen and fibronectin [30]. As a consequence of the inflammatory process, the expression of $\alpha_v\beta3$ is highly increased during angiogenesis [31–34]. In psoriasis, the

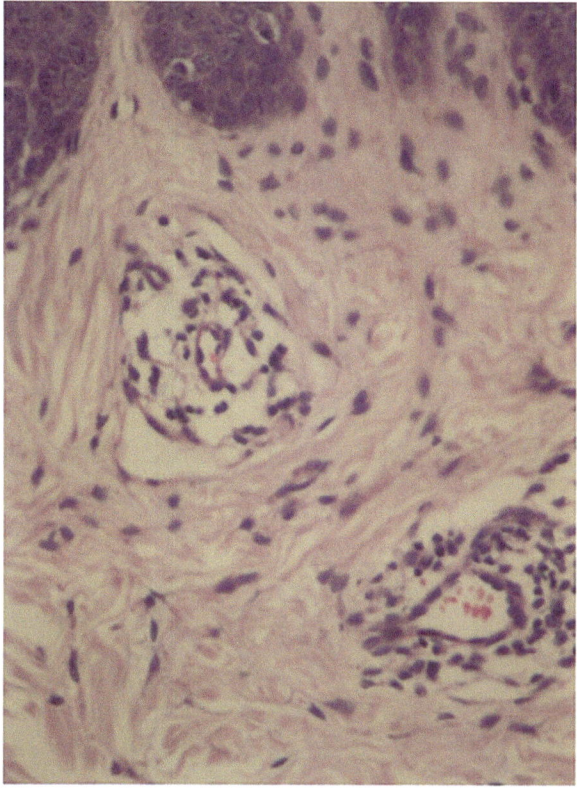

Fig. 3.10 Vascular proliferation and vasodilation in the superficial dermis. Archives of the Ambulatório de Psoríase, Pontifícia Universidade Católica de Campinas

expression of this integrin increases in endothelial cells compared to the skin of healthy individuals [35, 36].

Once angiogenesis is one of the main features of psoriasis, several studies have focused on the identification of pro-angiogenic mediators in the affected skin, which revealed a vast spectrum of factors, among which the vascular endothelial growth factor (VEGF), hypoxia inducible factors (HIFs), angiopoietins, the tumor necrosis factor (TNF), interleukins (IL-8, IL-17) and the transforming growth factor-β and α (TGF-β and TGF-α) [13, 37].

Vascular Endothelial Growth Factors (VEGF)

The development and activity of psoriasis are directly correlated to VEGF levels and their high-affinity receptors VEGFR-1 and VEGFR-2 [13, 14]. The active form of VEGF is a 40-45 kDa, homodimeric glycoprotein, described for the first time as a vascular permeability factor [13, 38].

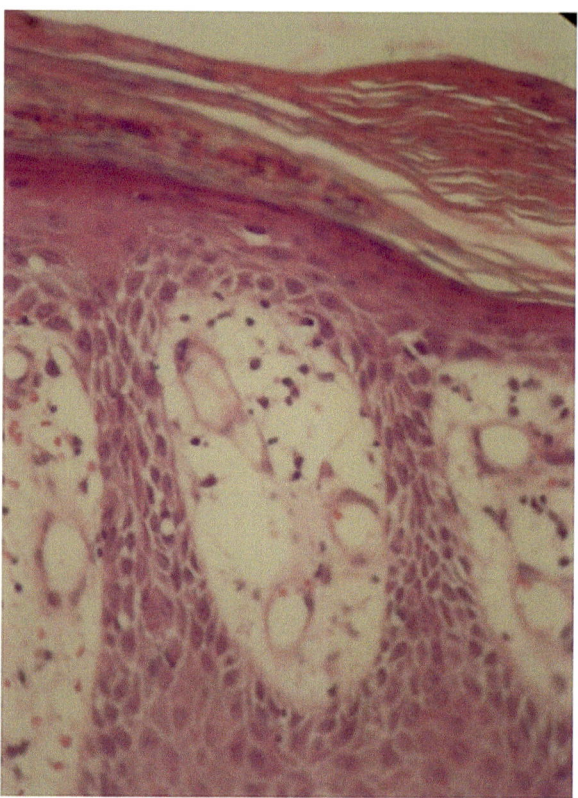

Fig. 3.11 In the superficial dermis, capillaries are increased in number and size, and show a tortuous appearance. Archives of the Ambulatório de Psoríase, Pontifícia Universidade Católica de Campinas

Twelve subtypes are known, seven of which show pro-angiogenic properties, and five anti-angiogenic action [39]. The gene encoding one of these subtypes, VEGF-A, is located near the PSORS1 gene (associated to the hereditary origin of psoriasis), both on chromosome 6p21 [40]. This gene is highly polymorphic, with some forms being associated to the early development of psoriasis [15]. Among the four isoforms (VEGF-A121, VEGF-A165, VEGF-A189, VEGF-A206), VEGF-A165 is the most common to stimulate angiogenesis [15] (Table 3.1).

VEGF can increase the expression of their own receptors on both keratinocytes and endothelial cells, which results in the activation of tyrosine kinase-mediated signal transduction pathways [15, 41–43]. One of these receptors, VEGFR-2, was shown to be highly associated to the proliferation, migration and the increased vascular permeability induced by VEGF [44].

The expression and secretion of skin VEGF-A by keratinocytes are triggered by the tumor growth factor (TGF)-α, found in high concentrations in patients with

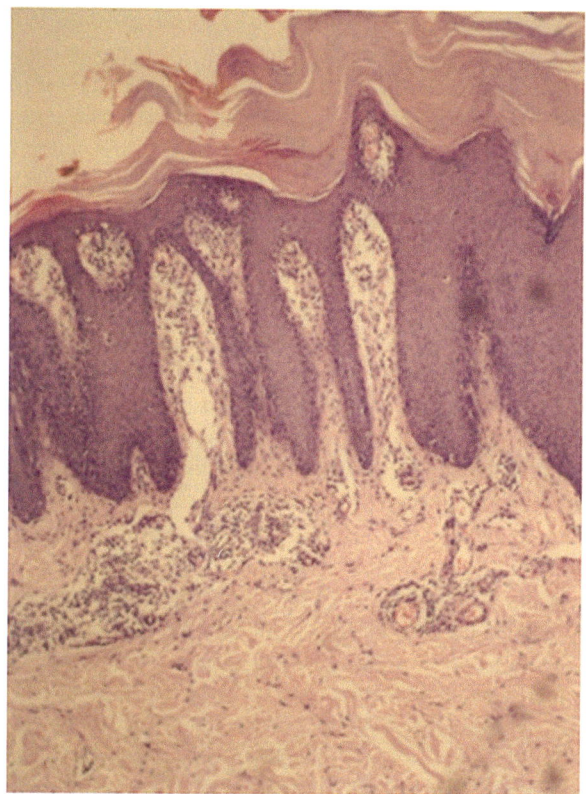

Fig. 3.12 Acanthosis, elongation of dermal papillae, hyperkeratosis with parakeratosis, and thinning of the suprapapillary region. Archives of the Ambulatório de Psoríase, Pontifícia Universidade Católica de Campinas

Table 3.1 VEGF-A

Isoforms	Functions	Secretion	High-affinity receptors[b]
VEGF-A121	1-increase vascular permeability	Keratinocyte stimulation by the tumor growth factor (TGF)-α and external skin trauma.	VEGFR-1
VEGF-A165[a]	2-control differentiation of endothelial cells		VEGFR-2
VEGF-A189	3-monocyte activation and chemotaxis		
VEGF-A206	4-keratinocyte proliferation.		

[a]More associated to angiogenic stimulation
[b]Expressed in keratinocytes and endothelial cells

psoriasis [15, 45]. Increases in the expression of VEGF m-RNA, VEGF-A itself and its high-affinity receptors, were demonstrated to occur in the epidermal keratinocytes and endothelial cells in the papillary dermis of sick patients [45].

In patients with psoriasis, the serum of both the affected and unaffected skin shows increased VEGF-A levels. Such an increase is correlated to disease severity and favors the early development of symptoms [46–48]. A study with transgenic mice expressing increased levels of VEGF demonstrated the development of psoriasis-like lesions, both clinically and histologically [49, 50]. These mice also remained healthy when treated with VEGF antagonists, corroborating the role of VEGF in the physiopathology of psoriasis [49, 50].

Case reports suggest that VEGF inhibitors, currently approved for the treatment of some tumors and ophthalmopathies, may improve the condition of patients with psoriasis [50]. Given the multifactor nature of this disorder, it is unlikely that VEGF inhibitors will be effective in all cases [50]. However, experimental data on the use of VEGF inhibitors in rats validate its importance for the treatment of particular cases [50].

When secreted physiologically, VEGF not only causes intense angiogenesis, but also contributes to the proliferation of keratinocytes and to the homeostasis of the epidermal layer, thus supporting skin recovery following acute disturbances [13]. Psoriasis may be also induced as a result of external trauma, a response known as the Koebner phenomenon. In addition, the disturbance of the skin barrier can induce simultaneous increases in VEGF concentrations in the skin [51].

Hypoxia Inducible Factors

The cardiovascular system provides both the oxygen and nutrients to tissues. When oxygen levels are reduced, a metabolic response is generated, with the release of Hypoxia Inducible Factors (HIFs) [13]. A physiological response is then triggered, resulting in angiogenesis. HIFs are composed of three α subunits (HIF-1α, HIF-2α, HIF-3α) and one β subunit (HIF-1β) [1].

HIF-1α is the most studied of them. An increase in its expression was observed under low oxygen concentrations, triggering the transcription of target genes associated to hypoxia [1].

Under physiological oxygen concentrations, α subunits are continually synthesized and expressed in the cytoplasm of lymphocytes. Its activity is controlled by degradation processes regulated by the proteasome, a complex of cytoplasmic and nuclear proteins capable of converting proteins into oligopeptides, with ATP consumption. The degradation occurs through the hydroxylation of the prolyl residues of α subunits by prolyl oxidases, which are only active under normal oxygen levels. The hydroxylated form is recognized by the Von Hippel-Lindau (VHL) tumor suppressor, and then finally enters the ubiquitin-proteasome pathway [52, 53].

Under hypoxia conditions, HIFs degradation is interrupted because of the inactivation of prolyl hydroxylases by oxygen reactive species [2]. As a result, HIF-α

subunits are not metabolized, leading to the phenomenon of nuclear translocation, in which angiogenesis-related genes are activated [54, 55].

HIFs have many gene targets, including different angiogenesis-regulating proteins: VEGF, angiopoeitins, VEGFR-1, VEGFR-2, IL-8 and Tie-2 [56–64].

An increased expression of those factors is observed in psoriatic lesions. This is probably due to the increase in the metabolic expenses resulting from epidermal proliferation, which leads to tissue hypoxia [1].

Angiopoietins

Angiopoietins (Ang-1 and Ang-2) are endogenous glycoproteins. Their binding to tyrosine kinase receptors (Tie-2) is crucial to the angiogenesis process [65–70]. Ang-1 and Ang-2 are antagonists.

Angiopoietin-1 induces the phosphorylation of the Tie-2 receptor, promoting the activation of an intracellular signal transduction cascade, which results in vessel remodeling and stabilization during angiogenesis [69] (Table 3.2). In embryogenesis, the formation of immature vessels is induced by VEGF. Here, angiogenesis depends on the interaction between VEGF and Angiopoietin-1 to be completed. In adult tissues, low levels of activated Tie-2 guarantee that the mature vascular endothelium remains at rest [71].

Angiopoietin-2, in turn, antagonizes the phosphorylation of the Tie-2 receptor, promoting vascular destabilization, which will lead to vascular regression in the absence of pro-angiogenic stimulation [13, 70] (Table 3.2).

It has been demonstrated that, during psoriasis, the Angiopoietin-Tie-2 system is activated in the papillary dermis [72, 73]. Endothelial cells express Angiopoietin-2, while Ang-1 is expressed by fibroblasts and mononuclear cells [72]. The reduction

Table 3.2 Angiopoetin's functions

	Function	Action on Tie-2 receptor	Expression sites
Angiopoietin-1	1. Vascular remodeling and stabilization. 2. Finishes the angiogenesis process.	Induces phosphorylation.	Fibroblasts and mononuclear cells.
Angiopoietin-2	1. Blocks angiogenic stimulation. 2. Vascular regression. 3. Sensitization of endothelial cells to inflammatory stimulation. 4. Leucocyte chemotaxis and adhesion.	Antagonizes phosphorylation.	Endothelial cells.

in Ang-2 expression, following adequate treatments, attests the importance of this glycoprotein in angiogenesis, and its relation to etiopathology of the disease [72].

In a study with transgenic mice expressing increased levels of the Tie-2 receptor, histological alterations similar to those of psoriasis were observed, such as epidermal hyperplasia, hyperkeratosis, parakeratosis, as well as an increase in dermal vascularization [73]. Suppressing this receptor expression completely reversed psoriasis [73].

Angiopoietin-2 is also capable of sensitizing endothelial cells to several inflammatory signals, facilitating leucocyte adhesion and chemotaxis, and contributing to inflammatory responses during the development of psoriasis [74].

Cytokines

Cytokines are also involved in angiogenesis, promoting the proliferation, elongation, increases in tortuosity and the dilation of capillaries. In addition, they also control the expression of other pro-inflammatory mediators, responsible for the development of psoriasis [13]. TNF, IL-8 and IL-17, pro-angiogenic cytokines acting on the physiopathology of psoriasis, are described as follows.

TNF

TNF-α is crucial to the development of psoriasis, once the use of anti-TNF drugs are highly effective [75]. TNF-α levels are increased in both the serum and lesioned skin of sick patients [76]. In lesioned skins, it is secreted by T-lymphocytes and antigen presenting cells [77]. This transmembrane protein is a precursor of several pro-inflammatory events, such as the activation of endothelial cells, resulting in the increased expression of adherence molecules and chemokines, keratinocyte stimulation for the production of other inflammatory mediators, and the activation of both macrophages and dendritic cells in the dermis [78]. Some of the pro-angiogenic factors induced by TNF-α are IL-8, VEGF and the fibroblast growth factor [79]. The impact of TNF on angiogenesis varies depending on its concentration and time of action, being also influenced by other factors, such as VEGF and the platelet activating factor [78, 80, 81]. The pre-formed TNF is stored in dermal mastocytes, and released following inflammatory stimulation [13]. Thus, TNF contributes to angiogenesis through direct stimulation, as well as inducing other pro-angiogenic factors [13].

IL-8

IL-8 is an 8.4 KDa, non-glycosylated protein, composed of two cysteine residues separated by a third amino acid. Its precursor belongs to the CXC chemokine family, and contains 99 amino acids [82]. It is secreted by monocytes, neutrophils, fibroblasts and endothelial cells, following stimulation by IL-1, TNF-α, IL-6, IFN-γ, lipopolysaccharides, oxygen reactive species and other mediators of cellular stress [13].

There are at least two types of specific receptors for IL-8 expressed by monocytes, neutrophils, fibroblasts, endothelial, mesothelial and tumor cells [13]. IL-8 binding to its receptors produces factors with both local and systemic effects, with inflammatory activity being directly related to their concentrations. This cytokine shows pro-angiogenic action and is highly expressed in several chronic inflammatory diseases, including psoriasis [83–85]. However, IL-8 angiogenic effect is independent of its pro-inflammatory activity, since it can stimulate angiogenesis without inflammation [84, 85]. It promotes chemotaxis and the activation of neutrophils and other inflammatory cells, as well as the migration, proliferation and formation of a tube of endothelial cells in vitro [83, 86–88]. This interleukin also inhibits the apoptosis of endothelial cells, stimulating anti-apoptotic proteins (Bcl-2), while inhibiting pro-apoptotic proteins (Bax) [88]. IL-8 and its m-RNA are found in high concentrations in psoriatic lesions, which will decrease following effective treatments [89]. In psoriasis, not only IL-8 induces angiogenesis, but also stimulates the proliferation of keratinocytes and other cells. In spite of these findings, studies reporting the efficiency of anti-IL-8 monoclonal antibodies as a treatment option are still lacking [13].

IL-17

Th17 lymphocytes secrete IL-17 after being stimulated by other cytokines (TGF-β, IL-6, IL-21 and IL-23) [13, 90]. The IL-17 cytokine family is formed of six members, IF-17 A-F, involved in inflammatory and autoimmune diseases, such as psoriasis [91]. Since the IL-17 cytokine family shares several receptors, different cellular targets are achieved during the inflammatory process [90]. The presence of m-RNAs of certain cytokines (IL-17A, IL-17F and IL-22) produced by Th17 lymphocytes in lesioned skins indicates the role these cells play on the pathogenesis of psoriasis [90]. IL-17A triggers the production of chemokines, growth factors and adhesion molecules by different types of cells, such as fibroblasts, epithelial and endothelial cells [13]. Some important cytokines produced are IL-6, IL-8, IL-1, G-CSF, GM-CSF and ICAM-1. IL-17 has pro-inflammatory potential, once it promotes neutrophil chemotaxis and induces granulopoiesis [13]. It also promotes the expression of TNF and IL-1β by human macrophages [92]. Studies with mice demonstrated IL-17A induces the formation of new vessels [93]. Part of IL-17A effect on angiogenesis could be explained by an increased expression of pro-angiogenic factors, including VEGF [13]. Recent studies demonstrated the efficacy of anti-IL17A treatments on patients with psoriasis, who showed important clinical improvements (83% of patients reached PASI 75 following 12 weeks of treatment) [90].

IL-9

Th2 and Th9 lymphocytes secrete IL-9, a cytokine that promotes the differentiation of Th17lymphocytes, thus resulting in the development of autoimmune and inflammatory diseases [94–96]. IL-9 is also secreted by Th17 lymphocytes; these latter are stimulated to produce IL-17 in vitro, in the presence of IL-9 [97–99]. The gene encoding IL-9 is located in the same chromosome region (5q31. 1) than those determining psoriasis susceptibility (5q31.1-q33.1) [13]. A study with transgenic rats indicated that IL-9 has an important role in the pathogenesis of psoriasis. Rats with the disease-associated phenotype showed increased levels of IL-9 and its receptors [13]. Intradermal injections of IL-9 were shown to trigger inflammatory processes with a Th17 response pattern, typical of psoriasis [100]. The study also showed this interleukin was associated to the angiogenic process and with increases in the expression of VEGF and CD31 [13]. The injection of anti-IL-9 antibodies in transgenic rats reduced not only the inflammatory process, but also angiogenesis. Therefore, IL-9 may be an important component in the development of psoriatic lesions, through the inflammatory and angiogenic activity of Th-17 lymphocytes [100].

Anti-angiogenic Drugs Used in the Treatment of Psoriasis

Cyclosporine

As previously mentioned, high concentrations of many potent angiogenic cytokines, such as TNF-alpha and IL-8, have been observed in psoriatic plaques. Increases in IL-8 were also shown to reduce the expression of thrombospondin-1, an anti-angiogenic protein, which confirms its role in the physiopathology of psoriasis [101].

Cyclosporine is an immunosuppressive drug that inhibits the activity of calcineurin-dependent nuclear transcription factors (NTFs) in activated T lymphocytes. Calcineurin is a cytoplasmic protein found in several cells producing inflammatory cytokines, which are involved in immune responses and in the activation of T-cells. Cyclosporine is also responsible for decreases in IL-1 and IL-8 levels in the epidermis of patients with psoriasis, where it suppresses keratinocyte hyperproliferation and dermal inflammation. This decrease in IL-8 levels allows a higher expression of thrombospondin-1, thereby inhibiting angiogenesis [101].

Cyclooxygenase (COX-2) is another mechanism through which cyclosporine inhibits angiogenesis. COX-2 is found in endothelial cells and inflammation sites, and catalyzes the conversion of arachidonic acid into prostaglandins, inflammation-inducing substances [102]. In psoriasis, the increase of pro-angiogenic factors, such as VEGF, stimulates the production of COX-2, which in turn activates T-cells and results in cutaneous inflammation. Cyclosporine inhibition is dose-dependent [102].

Fumarate Ester

Fumarate esters are derived from fumaric acid, a component of the Krebs cycle, and have been used for the treatment of psoriasis for over 30 years. These drugs show immune-modulating, anti-inflammatory and anti-proliferative properties, as well as apoptotic effects on T-cells [103]. Only dimethyl-fumarate exhibits anti-angiogenic activity (neither monomethyl-fumarate and fumaric acid do) [104].

Dimethyl-fumarate decreases SP1, a transcription factor known to promote angiogenesis and acting on VEGFR-2 receptors. When SP1 expression is prevented, these receptors are not activated and the production of VEGF and neo-vessels is subsequently impaired. In addition, patients with psoriasis are deficient in the production of endogenous fumarate, resulting in a higher production of hypoxia inducible factors (HIFs), especially HIF-1. HIF-1 induces the production of VEGF, even in the presence of normal oxygen tensions in cells. This process is inhibited when fumarate concentrations increase for there is no VEGF production [104].

Fumarate esters are safe, effective drugs, showing little toxicity [104].

Methotrexate

Methotrexate (MTX) is a folic acid analogue and a dihydrofolate reductase inhibitor, acting on the synthesis phase of cell cycles. Targets are, therefore, proliferating cell populations. In addition to its apoptotic effect on fast-dividing keratinocytes (seen in psoriasis), MTX also shows anti-inflammatory properties, decreasing the chemotaxis of polymorphonuclear cells, as well as an immunomodulatory action, diminishing the production of IL-1 and the density of Langerhans cells in the epidermis [105].

This well-established treatment reduces the expression of several adhesion molecules and cytokines, and shows anti-angiogenic activity, which prevents VEGF-induced neovascularization [106].

A significant reduction in the expression of VEGF is seen when MTX is used, both in psoriatic plaques, as well as in the surrounding skin. Mechanisms through which this drug inhibits angiogenesis include: direct effects on VEGF production by keratinocytes; indirect anti-proliferative activity, reducing the number of keratinocytes; the inhibition of cytokines such as IL-1 and TNF-alpha, potent angiogenic factors; and the modulation of adhesion molecules, such as integrins and selectins. The exact mechanism is still controversial and poorly investigated [106].

Acitretin

Acitretin is derived from retinoic acid, a vitamin A metabolite. It has been used in the treatment of psoriasis for its anti-proliferative activity, controlling both cell proliferation and differentiation. Applications include the treatment of other dermatological diseases where parakeratosis is observed, such as ichthyosis. Acitretin also suppresses the production of angiogenic factors, such as VEGF. The increase in VEGF levels in the blood and tissues results in the formation of dermal vessels, influencing the development and exacerbation of new psoriatic lesions. The suppression of vascular neoformation could thus be effective in the treatment of psoriasis [107].

In fact, the use of VEGF markers on skin fragments showed a reduction in VEGF following the treatment with acitretin, corroborating its anti-angiogenic action [107].

Anti-TNF Immunobiologicals – Infliximab, Adalimumab and Etanercept

Anti-TNF drugs have two effects – they reduce the inflammatory infiltrate and the activation of pro-inflammatory cytokines (decreasing TNF-alpha secretion by macrophages), while suppressing vascular proliferation [108].

TNF-alpha is one of the main pro-inflammatory cytokines involved in angiogenesis. Many reports show that cells stimulated by TNF-alpha may release angiogenesis-related cytokines, such as VEGF, Tie-2, BFGF, IL-8 and ICAM-1. In vivo, TNF-alpha increases VEGF expression, promoting the formation of morphologically altered vessels, as seen in psoriasis [108].

Treatments combining anti-TNF and anti-VEGF drugs were shown to be more efficient than the use of anti-VEGF drugs alone, evidencing the important role TNF-alpha plays in angiogenesis [108].

Anti IL-17A Immunobiologicals – Secukinumab

Drugs acting on specific immunological targets are increasing in importance as treatments of auto-immune diseases. Anti-IL-17A drugs are among the most promising [109].

CD4 T-lymphocytes are classified according to their cytokine production profile. The subtypes responsible for the physiopathology of psoriasis are TH1 and TH17 [109]. The production of IL-17 cytokine family and IL-22 is triggered by IL-23 in TH17 lymphocytes [109].

IL-17 is an angiogenic factor. It induces the production of IL-6, IL-8 and prostaglandins, and increases the expression of ICAM-1, an adhesion molecule secreted by fibroblasts and keratinocytes. Although it does not have a direct effect on the proliferation of endothelial vascular cells, IL-17 stimulates their migration and the production of capillary-like structures. This interleukin is also capable of stimulating VEGF production by fibroblasts. By inhibiting the activity of IL-17 and its derivatives, secukinumab inhibits angiogenesis indirectly [110].

Anti IL-12 AND Anti IL-23 Immunobiologicals – Ustekinumab

IL-12 and IL-23 stimulate the secretion of IL-17 and IL-22 by TH17 cells, resulting in the proliferation of keratinocytes and in dermal inflammation. Ustekinumab, a human monoclonal antibody, blocks angiogenesis indirectly. It acts on the p40 subunity of IL-12 and IL-23, reducing the production of IL-17 on psoriatic plaques.

Therefore, the production of VEGF and of other substances associated to vascular neoformation will be impaired [111].

Phototherapy

Phototherapy is an effective treatment for psoriasis. It suppresses the proliferation and induces the apoptosis of keratinocytes, in addition to regulating the activity of lymphocytes and antigen-presenting cells (APSs). If the production of cytokines such as TNF-alpha decreases because of reductions in VEGF expression by keratinocytes, angiogenesis will be also reduced [105]. Besides, with smaller numbers of keratinocytes, an indirect decrease in both the action and secretion of VEGF will be seen [105].

References

1. Torales-Cardeña A, Martínez-Torres I, Rodríguez-Martínez S, Gómez-Chávez, Cancino-Díaz JC, Vázquez-Sánchez E, et al. Cross talk between proliferative, angiogenic, and cellular mechanisms orchestred by HIF-1α in psoriasis. Mediators Inflamm. 2015;2015:607363.
2. Armstrong AW, Voyles SV, Armstrong EJ, Fuller EN, Rutledge JC. Angiogenesis and oxidative stress: common mechanisms linking psoriasis with atherosclerosis. J Dermatol Sci. 2011;63:1–9. Amsterdam: Elsevier.
3. Hertz A. Psoríase na infância. Revista Hospital Universitário Pedro Ernesto. Rio de Janeiro. 2014;13(Suppl 1):40–9.
4. Holubar K. Psoriasis – 100 years ago. Dermatology. 1900;180(1):1–4. Basel: Karger Publishers.
5. Holubar, K. Psoriasis and parapsoriasis: since 200 and 100 years, respectively. J Eur Acad Dermatol Venereol JEADV. 2003;17(2):126–7. England: Elsevier Science Publishers.
6. Romiti R, Maragno L, Arnone M, Takahashi MDF. Psoríase na infância e na adolescência. An Bras Dermatol. 2009;84(1):9–22. Rio de Janeiro: Sociedade Brasileira de Dermatologia.
7. Varrichi G, Granata F, Loffredo S, Genovese A, Marone G. Angiogenesis and lymphangiogenesis in inflammatory skin disorders. JAAD Case Rep. 2015;73(1):144–53. New York: Elsevier Inc.
8. Langley R, Krueger G, Griffiths C. Psoriasis: epidemiology, clinical features, and quality of life. Ann Rheum Dis. 2005;64(2):ii18–23. London: H.K. Lewis.
9. Parisi R, Symmons DP, Griffiths CE, Ashcroft DM. Global epidemiology of psoriasis: a systematic review of incidence and prevalence. J Invest Dermatol. 2013;133(2):377–85. Baltimore: Williams & Wilkins.
10. Enamandram M, Kimball AB. Psoriasis epidemiology: the interplay of genes and the environment. J Invest Dermatol. 2013;133:287–89. Baltimore: Williams & Wilkins.
11. Lupi O, Belo J, Cunha PR. Rotinas de Diagnóstico e Tratamento da Sociedade Brasileira de Dermatologia - SBD - 2ª Ed. Editora Guanabara Koogan, 2012. p. 680 ISBN: 9788581140841.
12. Murphy M, Kerr P, Grant-Kels JM. The histopathologic spectrum os psoriasis. Clin Dermatol. 2007;25:524–8.
13. Heidenreich R, Rocken M, Ghoreschi K. Angiogenesis drives psoriasis pathogenesis. Int J Exp Pathol; 2009;90:232–48. Oxford: Wiley.
14. Yamamoto T. Angiogenic and inflammatory properties of psoriatic arthritis. ISRN Dermatol. 2013;2013:630620. Cairo: Hindawi Pub. Corp.

15. Weidemann AK, Crawshaw AA, Byrne E, Young H. Vascular endothelial growth factor inhibitors: investigational therapies for the treatment of psoriasis. Clin Cosmet Investig Dermatol. 2013;6:233–44.Auckland: Dove Medical Press.
16. Creamer D, Allen MH, Sousa A, Poston R, Barker JN. Localization of endothelial proliferation and microvascular expansion in active plaque psoriasis. Br J Dermatol. 1997;136:859–65.
17. Telner P, Fekete Z. The capillary responses in psoriatic skin. J Invest Dermatol. 1961;36:225–30.
18. Ragaz A, Ackerman AB. Evolution, maturation, and regression of lesions of psoriasis. New observations and correlation of clinical and histologic findings. Am J Dermatopathol. 1979;1:199–214.
19. Braverman IM, Sibley J. Role of the microcirculation in the treatment and pathogenesis of psoriasis. J Invest Dermatol. 1982;78:12–7.
20. Kulka JP. Microcirculatory impairment as a factor in inflammatory tissue damage. Ann N Y Acad Sci. 1964;116:1018–44.
21. Hull SM, Goodfield M, Wood EJ, Cunliffe WJ. Active and inactive edges of psoriatic plaques: identification by tracing and investigation by laser-Doppler flowmetry and immunocytochemical techniques. J Invest Dermatol. 1989;92:782–5.
22. Goodfield M, Hull SM, Holland D, et al. Investigations of the 'active' edge of plaque psoriasis: vascular proliferation precedes changes in epidermal keratin. Br J Dermatol. 1994;131:808–13.
23. Bernhard JD. Clinical Pearl: Auspitz sign in psoriasis scale. JAAD Case Rep. 1997;36(4):621. New York: Elsevier Inc.
24. Výbohová D, Mellová Y, Adamicová K, Adamkov M, Hesková G. Quatitative comparison of angiogenesis and lymphangiogenesis in cutaneous lichen planus and psoriasis: Immunohistochemical assessment. Acta Histochemica. 2014;117(2015):20–8. Germany: Jena Gustav Fischer Verlag.
25. Zgraggen S, Huggenberger R, Kerl K, Detmar M. An important role of the SDF-1/CXCR4 axis in chronic skin inflammation. PLoS One. 2014;9(4):e93665. San Francisco: Public Library of Science.
26. Ghoreschi K, Thomas P, Breit S, et al. Interleukin-4 therapy of psoriasis induces Th2 responses and improves human autoimmune disease. Nat Med. 2003;9:40–6.
27. Ghoreschi K, Weigert C, Rocken M. Immunopathogenesis and role of T cells in psoriasis. Clin Dermatol. 2007;25:574–80.
28. Nickoloff BJ, Mitra RS, Varani J, Dixit VM, Polverini PJ. Aberrant production of interleukin-8 and thrombospondin-1 by psoriatic keratinocytes mediates angiogenesis. Am J Pathol. 1994;144:820–8.
29. Jin H, Varner J. Integrins: roles in cancer development and as treatment targets. Br J Cancer. 2004;90:561–5.
30. Cheresh DA. Human endothelial cells synthesize and express an Arg-Gly-Asp-directed adhesion receptor involved in attachment to fibrinogen and von Willebrand factor. Proc Natl Acad Sci U S A. 1987;84:6471–5.
31. Brooks PC, Clark RA, Cheresh DA. Requirement of vascular integrin alpha v beta 3 for angiogenesis. Science. 1994a;264:569–71.
32. Brooks PC, Montgomery AM, Rosenfeld M, et al. Integrin alpha v beta 3 antagonists promote tumor regression by inducing apoptosis of angiogenic blood vessels. Cell. 1994b;79:1157–64.
33. Kneilling M, Hultner L, Pichler BJ, et al. Targeted mast cell silencing protects against joint destruction and angiogenesis in experimental arthritis in mice. Arthritis Rheum. 2007;56:1806–16.
34. Muller-Hermelink N, Braumuller H, Pichler B, et al. TNFR1 signaling and IFN-gamma signaling determine whether T cells induce tumor dormancy or promote multistage carcinogenesis. Cancer Cell. 2008;13:507–18.
35. Creamer JD, Barker JN. Vascular proliferation and angiogenic factors in psoriasis. Clin Exp Dermatol. 1995;20:6–9.
36. Nickoloff BJ. Characterization of lymphocyte-dependent angiogenesis using a SCID mouse: human skin model of psoriasis. J Investig Dermatol Symp Proc. 2000;5:67–73.

37. Stinco G, Buligan C, Errichetti E, Valent F, Patrone P. Clinical and capillaroscopic modifications of the psoriatic plaque during therapy: observations with oral acitretin. Dermatol Res Pract. 2013;2013:781942. Cairo: Hindawi Pub. Corp.
38. Keck PJ, Hauser SD, Krivi G, et al. Vascular permeability factor, an endothelial cell mitogen related to PDGF. Science. 1989;246:1309–12.
39. Harper SJ, Bates DO. VEGF-A splicing: the key to anti-angiogenic therapeutics? Nat Rev Cancer. 2008;8:880–7.
40. Young HS, Summers AM, Read IR, et al. Interaction between genetic control of vascular endothelial growth factor production and retinoid responsiveness in psoriasis. J Invest Dermatol. 2006;126(2):453–9.
41. De Vries C, Escobedo JA, Ueno H, Houck K, Ferrara N, Wiliams LT. The fms-like tyrosine kinase, a receptor for vascular endothelial growth factor. Science. 1992;255:989–91.
42. Shibuya M. Role of VEGF-flt receptor system in normal and tumor angiogenesis. Adv Cancer Res. 1995;67:281–316.
43. Shibuya M, Claesson-Welsh L. Signal transduction by VEGF receptors in regulation of angiogenesis and lymphangiogenesis. Exp Cell Res. 2006;312:549–60.
44. Ferrara N, Gerber HP, LeCouter J. The biology of VEGF and its receptors. Nat Med. 2003;9:669–76.
45. Detmar M, Brown LF, Claffey KP, et al. Overexpression of vascular permeability factor/vascular endothelial growth factor and its receptors in psoriasis. J Exp Med. 1994;180:1141–6.
46. Creamer D, Allen M, Jaggar R, Stevens R, Bicknell R, Barker J. Mediation of systemic vascular hyperpermeability in severe psoriasis by circulating vascular endothelial growth factor. Arch Dermatol. 2002;138(6):791–6.
47. Bhushan M, McLaughlin B, Weiss JB, Griffiths CE. Levels of endothelial cell stimulating angiogenesis factor and vascular endothelial growth factor are elevated in psoriasis. Br J Dermatol. 1999;141:1054–60.
48. Nielsen HJ, Christensen IJ, Svendsen MN, et al. Elevated plasma levels of vascular endothelial growth factor and plasminogen activator inhibitor-1 decrease during improvement of psoriasis. Inflamm Res. 2002;51:563–7.
49. Detmar M, Brown LF, Schon MP, et al. Increased microvascular density and enhanced leukocyte rolling and adhesion in the skin of VEGF transgenic mice. J Invest Dermatol. 1998;111:1–6.
50. Xia YP, Li B, Hylton D, Detmar M, Yancopoulos GD, Rudge JS. Transgenic delivery of VEGF to mouse skin leads to an inflammatory condition resembling human psoriasis. Blood. 2003;102:161–8.
51. Elias PM, Arbiser J, Brown BE, et al. Epidermal vascular endothelial growth factor production is required for permeability barrier homeostasis, dermal angiogenesis, and the development of epidermal hyperplasia: implications for the pathogenesis of psoriasis. Am J Pathol. 2008;173:689–99.
52. Hon W-C, Wilson MI, Harlos K, et al. Structural basis for the recognition of hydroxyproline in HIF-1α by pVHL. Nature. 2002;417(6892):975–8.
53. Min JH, Yang H, Ivan M, Gertler F, Kaelin Jr WG, Pavietich NP. Structure of an HIF-1alpha-pVHL complex: hydroxyproline recognition in signaling. Science. 2002;296(5574):1886–9.
54. Li Y-N, Xi M-M, Guo Y, Hai C-X, Yang W-L, Qin X-J. NADPH oxidase-mitochondria axis-derived ROS mediate arsenite-inducedHIF-1alpha stabilization by inhibiting prolyl hydroxylases activity. Toxicol Lett. 2014;224(2):165–74.
55. Acker T, Fandrey J, Acker H. The good, the bad and the ugly in oxygen-sensing: ROS, cytochromes and prolylhydroxylases. Cardiovasc Res. 2006;71(2):195–207.
56. Levy AP, Levy NS, Wegner S, Goldberg MA. Transcriptional regulation of the rat vascular endothelial growth factor gene by hypoxia. J Biol Chem. 1995;270:13333–40.
57. Liu Y, Cox SR, Morita T, Kourembanas S. Hypoxia regulates vascular endothelial growth factor gene expression in endothelial cells. Identification of a 5′ enhancer. Circ Res. 1995;77:638–43.

58. Forsythe JA, Jiang BH, Iyer NV, et al. Activation of vascular endothelial growth factor gene transcription by hypoxia-inducible factor 1. Mol Cell Biol. 1996;16:4604–13.
59. Takeda N, Maemura K, Imai Y, et al. Endothelial PAS domain protein 1 gene promotes angiogenesis through the transactivation of both vascular endothelial growth factor and its receptor, Flt-1. Circ Res. 2004;95:146–53.
60. Elvert G, Kappel A, Heidenreich R, et al. Cooperative interaction of hypoxia inducible factor (HIF)-2a and Ets-1 in the transcriptional activation of vascular endothelial growth factor receptor-2 (Flk-1). J Biol Chem. 2003;278:7520–30.
61. Kim KS, Rajagopal V, Gonsalves C, Johnson C, Kalra VK, et al. A novel role of hypoxia-inducible factor in cobalt chloride- and hypoxia-mediated expression of IL-8 chemokine in human endothelial cells. J Immunol. 2006;177:7211–24.
62. Tian H, McKnight SL, Russell DW. Endothelial PAS domain protein 1 (EPAS1), a transcription factor selectively expressed in endothelial cells. Genes Dev. 1997;11:72–82.
63. Chen Y, Zhang L, Pan Y, Ren X, Hao Q, Over-expression of semaphorin4d, hypoxia-inducible factor-1α and vascular endothelial growth factor is related to poor prognosis in ovarian epithelial cancer. Int J Mol Sci. 2012;13(10):13264–74.
64. Nikitenko LL, Smith DM, Bicknell R, Rees MCP. Transcriptional regulation of the CRLR gene in human microvascular endothelial cells by hypoxia. FASEB J. 2003;17(11):1499–501.
65. Bisht M, Dhasmana DC, Bist SS. Angiogenesis: Future of pharmacological modulation. Indian J Pharmacol. 2010;42:2–8. Mumbai: Medknow Publications.
66. Dumont DJ, Gradwohl G, Fong GH, et al. Dominant-negative and targeted null mutations in the endothelial receptor tyrosine kinase, tek, reveal a critical role in vasculogenesis of the embryo. Genes Dev. 1994;8:1897–909.
67. Sato TN, Tozawa Y, Deutsch U, et al. Distinct roles of the receptor tyrosine kinases Tie-1 and Tie-2 in blood vessel formation. Nature. 1995;376:70–4.
68. Davis S, Aldrich TH, Jones PF, et al. Isolation of angiopoietin-1, a ligand for the TIE2 receptor, by secretion-trap expression cloning. Cell. 1996;87:1161–9.
69. Suri C, Jones PF, Patan S, Bartunkova S, Maisonpierre PC, Davis S, Sato TN, et al. Requisite role of angiopoietin-1, a ligand for the TIE2 receptor, during embryonic angiogenesis. Cell. 1996;87:1171–80.
70. Maisonpierre PC, Suri C, Jones PF, et al. Angiopoietin-2, a natural antagonist for Tie2 that disrupts in vivo angiogenesis. Science. 1997;277:55–60.
71. Wong AL, Haroon ZA, Werner S, Dewhirst MW, Greenberg CS, Peters KG. Tie2 expression and phosphorylation in angiogenic and quiescent adult tissues. Circ Res. 1997;81:567–74.
72. Kuroda K, Sapadin A, Shoji T, Fleischmajer R, Lebwohl M. Altered expression of angiopoietins and Tie2 endothelial receptor in psoriasis. J Invest Dermatol. 2001;116:713–20.
73. Voskas D, Jones N, Van Slyke P, et al. A cyclosporine-sensitive psoriasis-like disease produced in Tie2 transgenic mice. Am J Pathol. 2005;166:843–55.
74. Fiedler U, Reiss Y, Scharpfenecker M, et al. Angiopoietin-2 sensitizes endothelial cells to TNF-alpha and has a crucial role in the induction of inflammation. Nat Med. 2006;12:235–9.
75. Sato K, Takaishi M, Tokuoka S, Sano S. Involvement of TNF-α converting enzyme in the development of psoriasis-like lesions in a mouse model. PLoS One. 2014;9(11):e112408. San Francisco: Public Library of Science.
76. Zaba LC, Cardinale I, Gilleaudeau P, Sullivan-Whalen M, Suárez-Fariñas M, Fuentes-Duculan J, et al. Amelioration of epidermal hyperplasia by TNF inhibition is associated with reduced Th17 responses. J Exp Med. 2007;204(13):3183–94.
77. Yost J, Gudjonsson JE. The role of TNF inhibitors in psoriasis therapy: new implications for associated comorbidities. F1000 Med Rep. 2009;1:30.
78. Patterson C, Perrella MA, Endege WO, Yoshizumi M, Lee ME, Haber E. Downregulation of vascular endothelial growth factor receptors by tumor necrosis factor-alpha in cultured human vascular endothelial cells. J Clin Invest. 1996;98:490–6.
79. Yoshida S, Ono M, Shono T, et al. Involvement of interleukin-8, vascular endothelial growth factor, and basic fibroblast growth factor in tumor necrosis factor alpha-dependent angiogenesis. Mol Cell Biol. 1997;17:4015–23.

80. Fajardo LF, Kwan HH, Kowalski J. Dual role of tumor necrosis factor-alpha in angiogenesis. Am J Pathol. 1992;140:539–44.
81. Montrucchio G, Lupia E, Battaglia E, et al. Tumor necrosis factor alpha-induced angiogenesis depends on in situ platelet-activating factor biosynthesis. J Exp Med. 1994;180:377–82.
82. Qazi BS, Tang K, Qazi A. Recent advances in underlying pathologies provide insight into interleukin-8 expression-mediated inflammation and angiogenesis. Int J Inflam. 2011;2011: Article ID 908468, 13 pages.
83. Koch AE, Polverini PJ, Kunkel SL, et al. Interleukin-8 as a macrophage-derived mediator of angiogenesis. Science. 1992;258:1798–801.
84. Strieter RM, Kunkel SL, Elner VM, et al. Interleukin-8. A corneal factor that induces neovascularization. Am J Pathol. 1992;141:1279–84.
85. Hu DE, Hori Y, Fan TP. Interleukin-8 stimulates angiogenesis in rats. Inflammation. 1993;17:135–43.
86. Man XY, Yang XH, Cai SQ, Yao YG, Zheng M. Immunolocalization and expression of vascular endothelial growth factor receptors (VEGFRs) and neuropilins (NRPs) on keratinocytes in human epidermis. Mol Med. 2006;12:127–36.
87. Shono T, Ono M, Izumi H, et al. Involvement of the transcription factor NF-kappaB in tubular morphogenesis of human microvascular endothelial cells by oxidative stress. Mol Cell Biol. 1996;16:4231–9.
88. Li A, Dubey S, Varney ML, Dave BJ, Singh RK. IL-8 directly enhanced endothelial cell survival, proliferation, and matrix metalloproteinases production and regulated angiogenesis. J Immunol. 2003;170:3369–76.
89. Ghoreschi K, Rocken M. Molecular and cellular basis for designing gene vaccines against inflammatory autoimmune disease. Trends Mol Med. 2003;9:331–8.
90. Raychaudhuri SP. Role of IL-17 in psoriasis and psoriatic arthritis. Clin Rev Allergy Immunol. 2013;44(2):183–93. Totowa: Humana Press.
91. Kolls JK, Linden A. Interleukin-17 family members and inflammation. Immunity. 2004;21:467–76.
92. Jovanovic DV, Di Battista JA, Martel-Pelletier J, et al. IL-17 stimulates the production and expression of proinflammatory cytokines, IL-beta and TNF-alpha, by human macrophages. J Immunol. 1998;160:3513–21.
93. Numasaki M, Fukushi J, Ono M, et al. Interleukin-17 promotes angiogenesis and tumor growth. Blood. 2003;101:2620–7.
94. Goswami R, Kaplan MH. A brief history of IL-9. J. Immunol. 2011;186(6):3283–8. Rockville: The American Association of Immunologists, Inc.
95. Nowak EC, Weaver CT, Turner H, Begum-Haque S, Schreiner B, Coyle AJ, et al. IL-9 as a mediator of Th17-driven inflammatory disease. J Exp Med. 2009;206(8):1653–60. Rockefeller: The Rockefeller University Press.
96. Li H, Nourbakhsh B, Ciric B, Zhang GX, Rostami A. Neutralization of IL-9 ameliorates experimental autoimmune encephalomyelitis by decreasing the effector T cell population. J Immunol. 2010;185:4095–100. Rockville: The American Association of Immunologists, Inc.
97. Beriou G, Bradshaw EM, Lozano E, Costantino CM, Hastings WD, Orban T, et al. TGF-beta induces IL-9 production from human Th17 cells. J Immunol. 2010;185:46–54. Rockville: The American Association of Immunologists, Inc.
98. Noelle RJ, Nowak EC. Cellular sources and immune functions of interleukin-9. Nat Rev Immunol. 2010;10:683–7. London: Nature Pub Group.
99. Elyaman W, Bradshaw EM, Uyttenhove C, Dardalhon V, Awasthi A, Imitola J, et al. IL-9 induces differentiation of TH17 cells and enhances function of FoxP3+ natural regulatory T cells. Proc Natl Acad Sci U S A 2009; vol 106: 12885–12890. doi: 10.1073/pnas.0812530106 15-27. Washington: National Academy of Sciences.
100. Singh TP, Schön MP, Wallbrecht K, Gruber-Wackernagel A, Wang XJ, Wolf P. Involvement of IL-9 in Th17-associated inflammation and angiogenesis of psoriasis. PLoS One. 2013;8(1):e51752. San Francisco: Public Library of Science.

101. Heenan PJ, Skender-Kalnenas TM. Cyclosporine and angiogenesis in psoriasis. J Am Acad Dermatol. 1996. 35(6): 1019–20. St. Louis: Mosby.
102. Hernández GL, Volpert OV, Íñiguez MA, Lorenzo E, Martínez-Martínez S, Grau R et al. Selective inhibition of vascular endothelial growth factor–mediated angiogenesis by cyclosporin a: roles of the nuclear factor of activated T cells and cyclooxygenase 2. J Exp Med. 2001. 193(5):607–20. New York: Rockefeller University Press.
103. Sociedade Brasileira de Dermatologia. Consenso Brasileiro de Psoríase 2012 – Guias de avaliação e tratamento. 2 ed. Rio de Janeiro: Sociedade Brasileira de Dermatologia; 2009.
104. Arbiser JL. Fumarate esters as angiogenesis inhibitors: key to action in psoriasis. J Invest Dermatol. 2011;131(6):1189–91. Baltimore: Williams & Wilkins.
105. Martins GA, Arruda L. Tratamento sistêmico da psoríase – Parte I: metotrexato e acitretina. An Bras Dermatol. 2004. 79(3):263–78. Rio de Janeiro: Sociedade Brasileira de Dermatologia.
106. Shaker GO, Khairallah M, Rasheed HM, Abdel-Halim MR, Abuzeid, OM, El Tawdi HH, el al. Antiangiogenic effect of methotrexate and puva on psoriasis. Cell Biochem Biophys. 2013;67(2):735–42. Totowa: Humana Press.
107. Kim CY, Kim SM, Kim GD. The effect of acitretin to the expression of vascular endothelial growth factor in psoriasis. J Life Sci. 2009;19(3):327–33. Korea: Korean Society of Life Science.
108. Liu Y, Yang G, Zhang J, Xing K, Dai L, Cheng L et al. Anti-TNF-alpha monoclonal antibody reverses psoriasis through dual inhibition of inflammation and angiogenesis. Int Immunopharmacol. 2015;28:731–43. New York: Elsevier Science.
109. Raychaudhuri SP. Role of IL-17 in psoriasis and psoriatic arthritis. Clin Rev Allergy Immunol. 2013;44:183–93. Totowa: Humana Press.
110. Numasaki M, Fukushi J, Ono M, Narula SK, Zavodny PJ, Kudo T, et al. Interleukin-17 promotes angiogenesis and tumor growth. Blood Res. 2003;101(7):2620–7. Seoul: Korean Society of Hematology.
111. Golmia RP, Martins AHB, Scheinberg M. Quando anti-TNF não obtém sucesso, anti-IL-12-23 é opção alternativa na psoríase e na artrite psoriásica. Rev Bras Reumatol. 2014;54(3):247–9. Rio de Janeiro: Elsevier Editora Ltda.

Angiogenesis and Nonmelanoma Skin Cancer

4

Omer Ibrahim and Sherrif F. Ibrahim

Introduction

Basal cell carcinoma (BCC) and squamous cell carcinoma (SCC) are the two most common types of cutaneous neoplasms [1]. The worldwide incidence of nonmelanoma skin cancer (NMSC) has increased by 3–8% every year, and the incidence in the US may increase by 50% by the year 2030 [2–4]. In order to treat these tumors, especially in their aggressive forms not amenable to surgery, an understanding of their pathogenesis is integral. A multitude of factors interact with one another to promote tumorigenesis and tumor survival. This chapter will discuss the pathogenesis of BCC and SCC, with particular emphasis on how aberrant angiogenesis promotes tumor progression, and will elucidate nonsurgical treatment modalities, both old and new, that directly or indirectly target angiogenesis in their anti-proliferative actions.

Basal Cell Carcinoma

Pathogenesis

BCC is the most common skin cancer, comprising about 80% of NMSC [5]. BCC arises from the cells of the basal layer of the epidermis and hair follicles [6]. The pathogenesis and proliferation of this tumor is a multifactorial process that

O. Ibrahim, MD
Department of Dermatology, Cleveland Clinic Foundation, Cleveland, OH, USA
e-mail: ibrahio@ccf.org

S.F. Ibrahim, MD, PhD (✉)
Assistant Professor, Department of Dermatology, Division of Dermatologic Surgery,
Wilmot Cancer Center, University of Rochester, 400 Red Creek Drive, Suite 200,
Rochester, NY, 14623, USA
e-mail: sherrif_ibrahim@urmc.rochester.edu

© Springer-Verlag London Ltd. 2017
J.L. Arbiser (ed.), *Angiogenesis-Based Dermatology*,
DOI 10.1007/978-1-4471-7314-4_4

eventually leads to cellular proliferation and differentiation, tumor survival, and angiogenesis (Fig. 4.1, Table 4.1). In recent years, cancer genetics have elucidated the role epidermal growth factor receptor (EGFR) activation in the development of BCC [7]. EGFR appears to be mutated, dysregulated, or over-expressed in many cancers, including BCC [7]. As a result, mutated or over-expressed EGFR leads to impaired immune response in human skin and promotion of cellular proliferation, differentiation, and survival [8].

In addition to EGFR signaling, established research has shown that the Hedgehog (Hh) signaling pathway is the predominant player in the tumorigenesis of BCC (Fig. 4.2) [7]. The Hh pathway is quiescent and nonfunctional in mature skin. It is composed of patched-1 (PTCH), a transmembrane receptor, which normally exerts an inhibitory effect on smoothened (SMO), a transmembrane protein. When PTCH is dysfunctional, it cannot apply its normal inhibitory effect on SMO. In its unregulated active form, SMO promotes cellular replication and ultimately, tumor development. The majority of BCC carry a mutation in the PTCH-1 resulting in inactive PTCH-1, while a minority carry a mutation in the SMO gene resulting in overexpression of the Hh pathway [7].

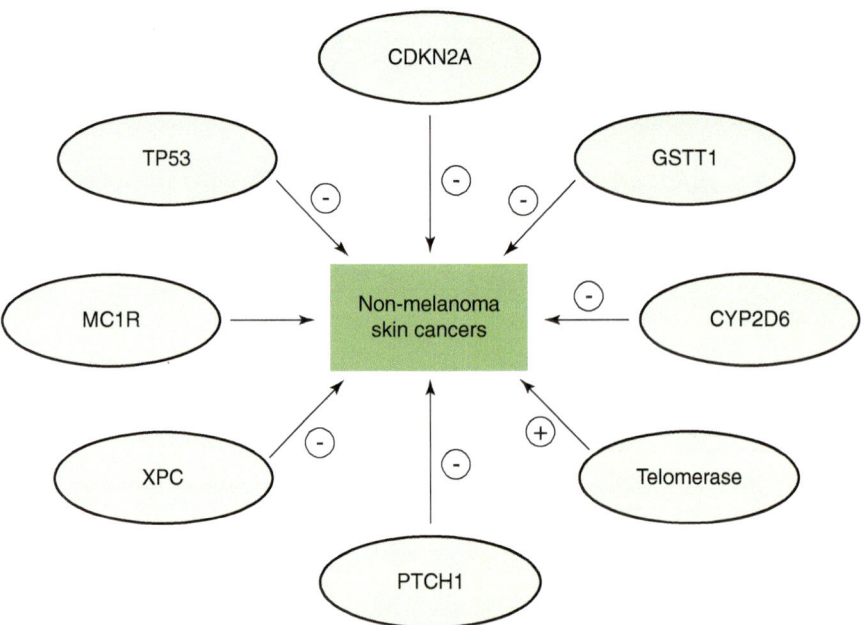

Fig. 4.1 Major pathways involved in the pathogenesis of non-melanoma skin cancers. *CDKN2A* cyclin-dependent kinase inhibitor 2A, *GSTT1* glutathione S-transferase theta 1, *CYP2D6* cytochrome P450, family 2, subfamily D, polypeptide 6, *PTCH1* patched homolog 1, *XPC* xeroderma pigmentosum, complementation group C, *MC1R* melanocortin 1 receptor, *TP53* tumour protein 53 (Adapted with permission from Madan et al. [47])

Table 4.1 Environmental risk factors for non-melanoma skin cancers

	Type of non-melanoma skin cancer
Solar UV radiation	BCC, SCC
Human papillomavirus	SCC, BCC
Iatrogenic immunosuppression	SCC, BCC
HIV/AIDS and non-Hodgkin lymphoma	BCC, SCC
PUVA therapy	SCC, BCC
Photosensitising drugs (e.g., fluoroquinolone antibiotics)	SCC, BCC
UVB radiation	BCC
Ionising radiation	BCC
Occupational factors	BCC, SCC
Arsenic	SCC, BCC
Tobacco smoking	SCC

Adapted with permission from Madan et al. [47]
UV ultraviolet, *BCC* basal-cell carcinoma, *SCC*=squamous-cell carcinoma, *PUVA* psoralen and UVA.

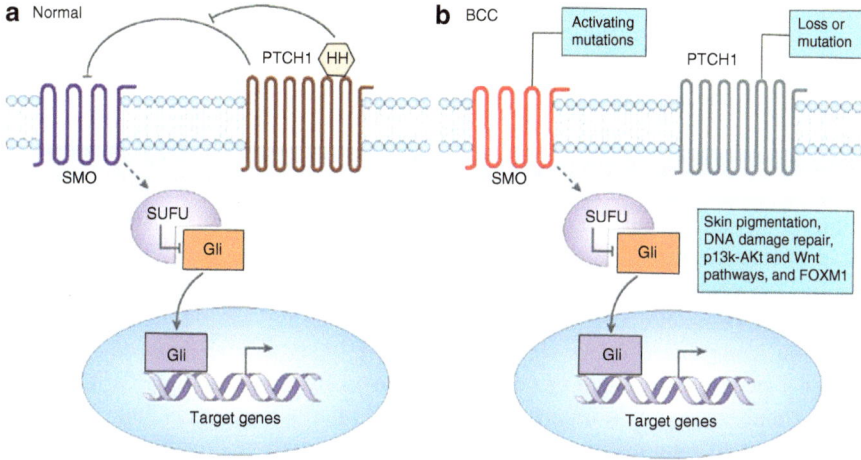

Fig. 4.2 The Hedgehog (*HH*) signaling pathway. (**a**) Normally, patched 1 (*PTCH 1*) inhibits smoothened (*SMO*). Sonic hedgehog (*SHH*) can bind to the PTCH 1 receptor, thereby relieving the inhibition of SMO by PTCH1; SMO then sends signals through a series of interacting proteins, including suppressor of fused (*SUFU*), resulting in activation of the downstream Gli family of transcription factors (GLI1, GLI2 and GLI3). (**b**) Sporadic BCCs routinely carry mutations in *PTCH1* and *TP53,* and, in 10% of instances, in *SMO*. Other mutations implicated in BCC development include genes that regulate skin color, DNA damage repair genes, members of the phosphoinositide 3-kinase (*PI3K*)–Akt and the Wnt pathways and FOXM1 (Adapted with permission from: Epstein [48])

In addition to promoting the proliferation and differentiation of adult stem cells, the Hh signaling pathway has also been shown to be a key mediator of angiogenesis and likely tumor survival [9]. In early embryonic development, the Hh pathway plays a normal role in angiogenesis. It has been shown that this pathway induces the expression of vascular endothelial growth factors (VEGFs) and migration of endothelial cells [9]. The Hh pathway also leads to a signaling cascade that ultimately aids in coronary and pulmonary angiogenesis [10, 11]. In post-natal life, reports have shown that in ischemic or injured tissue, Hh expression is increased, playing a role in regeneration, repair, and survival [12]. Therefore in an aberrant, over-expressed state such as in BCC, Hh signaling may lead to unregulated angiogenesis and tumor survival [13].

Treatment

Although surgical excision remains the gold standard for the treatment of BCC, patients who are poor surgical candidates or with metastatic BCC may not be amenable to surgical intervention. Therefore, research has brought to the forefront several alternative modalities in the treatment of BCC that among many other mechanisms, retard tumor growth, oftentimes acting on its angiogenic properties. The most exciting development in the treatment of BCC has been the development of oral Hh inhibitors. The first of these to come to market, vismodegib (Erivedge, Genentech Roche) was recently approved for the treatment of locally advanced or metastatic disease. As previously mentioned, when PTCH-1 is dysfunctional, it fails to exert its normal inhibitory effect on SMO, leading to overexpression of SMO and cellular proliferation (Fig. 4.2). Vismoedgib specifically acts as a SMO inhibitor, thus acting at a downstream point in the Hh pathway and having efficacy whether tumors harbor mutations in PTCH-1 or SMO. In a Phase I trial of 33 patients with refractory advanced or metastasized BCC, there was an overall 58% response, either partial or complete, and the duration of response was 12.8 months and ongoing; several reports have shown similar results [14]. Other well-established drugs have been experimentally employed in the treatment of BCC, such as the EGFR-inhibitor cetuximab. In one case report, an 87-year-old man with giant, nodular mid-facial BCC showed minimal progression over 4 months with treatment with cetuximab [15]. In another case of two palliative patients, tumor stability was noted with cetuximab, and one patient developed liver metastases following cessation of treatment [16]. Finally, a case series reported that when four patients with BCC were treated with cetuximab, two had complete remission and two had partial remission; three patients relapsed after treatment cessation [17].

In addition to systemic therapy, several topical modalities have been trialed in the treatment of BCC. 5-fluorouracil (5-FU) 5% cream is approved by the US Food and Drug Administration (FDA) clearance rate in lesions after twice a day application for 8–12 weeks [18]. In addition to 5-FU, imiquimod, a topical immunomodulator, has been successfully used in the treatment of BCC. Imiquimod 5.0% cream is US FDA approved to treat nonfacial superficial BCC [19]. Once daily application,

5-days per week for 6–12 weeks leads to the highest clearance rate of lesions (up to 80%) [18]. This topical drug activates toll-like receptor 7 (TLR 7) [19]. TLR 7 is subsequently responsible for the upregulation of many different cytokines, including interferon-α (IFN-α), tumor necrosis factor-α (TNF-α) and interleukin-12 (IL-12) (Fig. 4.3) [20]. The role of Type 1 interferons (IFNs) in the apoptosis and anti-angiogenesis of BCC cannot be understated.

IFNs are naturally occurring glycoproteins that are secreted by cells in response to biologic stimuli, including viral infection [21]. Since their discovery, research has elucidated their anti-viral, anti-proliferative, and immunomodulatory properties [22]. Type I IFNs (IFN-α/β) have been shown to have an anti-proliferative, prodifferentiation effect on normal keratinocytes. Keratinocytes supplemented with Type 1 IFNs exhibited an average of 70% growth inhibition, as well as terminal differentiation. Several reports have demonstrated the effect of Type 1 IFNs on antiangiogenesis. Mouse IFNs α/β have been shown to impair wound healing in mice by inhibiting the endothelial and epidermal cell proliferation [23]. Another study showed that mice implanted with IFN α/β and proangiogenic factors such as VEGF demonstrated a significantly less number of blood vessels than the mice without IFN α/β [24]. Moreover, the immunomodulatory effects of Type 1 IFNs have been explained by experiments that have demonstrated the induction of class I major histocompatibility (MCH) antigen expression in keratinocytes treated with Type 1 IFNs [25]. Through these innovations, the mechanism by which imiquimod may play a role in the destruction of BCC has been elucidated.

In addition, IFN-α has been explored as a direct treatment for BCC. One group demonstrated that IFN-α demonstrated growth inhibitory effects on primary BCC cell lines in vitro [26]. In another study of 15 patients with BCC, treatment with IFN-α led to the expression of CD95 and CD95L, which ultimately led to cell death by suicide and fratricide [27]. In one report, four patients with nodular BCC were treated with intralesional IFN-α and demonstrated resolution of the BCC on histopathologic examination [28]. A similar study demonstrated that in six patients with nodular and superficial BCC treated with intralesional IFN-α, two BCCs were cured and four showed clinical and histologic signs of improvement [29]. Given its anti-proliferative, anti-angiogenic, and immunomodulatory properties, IFN-α therapy may be a plausible option in the treatment of patients who are poor surgical candidates, or in order to shrink tumor size prior to surgery.

Squamous Cell Carcinoma

Pathogenesis

SCC is the second most common cutaneous neoplasm, after BCC. As in the development of BCC, the pathogenesis of SCC is a multifactorial and multistage process that occurs gradually over time in response to chronic ultra-violet (UV) radiation exposure (Fig. 4.1, Table 4.1). In 1928, Findlay was the first to describe that chronic UV radiation could induce SCC in mice [30]. During the initial phases of UV-induced

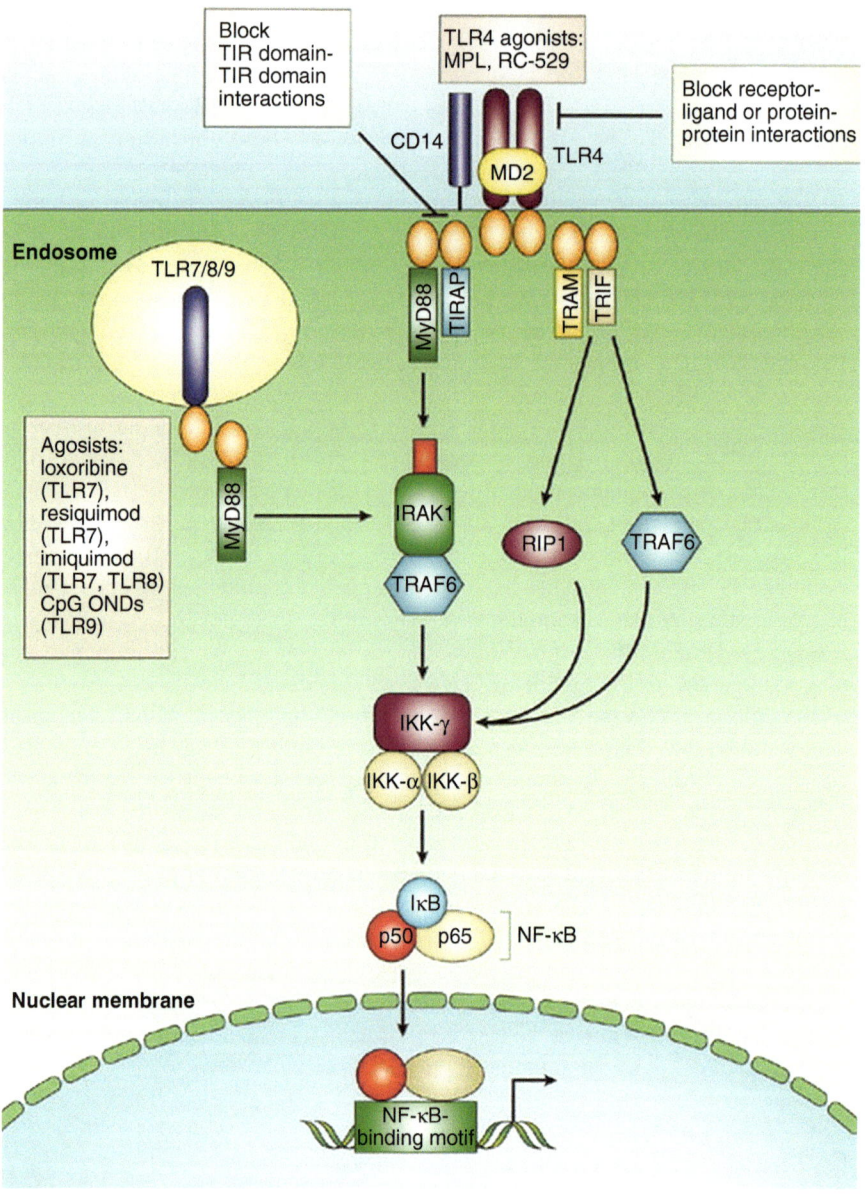

Fig. 4.3 Imiquimod signaling pathway, as part of a complex interation of toll-like receptors (*TLRs*) and the immune system. Imiquimod acts upon TLR7 within the cellular endosome, which in turn interacts with a cytoplasmic adaptor receptor, MyD88. MyD88 mediates the association with the serine-threonine kinase, IRAK. This in turn leads to the ultimate activation of nuclear factor-κB (*NF-κB*) and synthesis of numerous Type I interferons (Adapted with permission from Ulevitch [49])

damage, keratinocytes undergo point mutations. Nearly 60% of SCC demonstrates mutations in the p53 tumor suppressor gene [31]. UV-induced mutations in p53 impair its normal ability to activate DNA repair enzymes, arrest the cell cycle, and induce cellular apoptosis, leading to aberrant cellular proliferation and tumor development [32]. Once tumorigenesis has initiated, a multitude of factors interplay to support tumor growth and survival. One such key factor in the development of SCC, and to a lesser extent BCC, is the increased expression of the enzyme cyclooxygenase-2 (COX-2) in the epidermis. COX-2 is integral in the formation of prostaglandins, potent mediators of inflammation, angiogenesis, and immunosuppression (Figs. 4.4 and 4.5) [33]. In preclinical studies, mice that were deficient in COX-2 exhibited significantly less numbers of SCC than wild-type mice, and in a clinical trial by Elmets and colleagues, patients treated with celecoxib, a COX-2 inhibitor, exhibited significantly fewer NMSC than patients treated with placebo [34, 35]. Furthermore, the formation of reactive oxygen intermediates promotes DNA damage and tumor progression [32]. Finally, as in BCC, SCC, especially of the head and neck, demonstrate overexpression of EGFR, leading to signal transduction that induces carcinogenesis [36].

Treatment

In the last decade or so, much investigation and ongoing research have sought to investigate the non-surgical treatment of advanced SCC, especially of the head and neck. Some of these investigational treatments target the angiogenic properties of SCC, among a multitude of interplaying mechanisms in anti-carcinogenesis. The EGFR inhibitor cetuximab has shown such potential in the treatment of locally advanced, metastatic, and recurrent SCC of the head and neck, that it has become the only targeted EGFR inhibitor to receive FDA clearance for use in localized disease concomitantly with radiation [37]. In one randomized study, patients with locally advanced SCC of the head and neck treated with cetuximab and radiation demonstrated an overall response rate of 74% in contrast to 64% in patients treated with radiotherapy alone [38]. Also, studies have shown that cetuximab in combination with platinum based chemotherapy and 5-fluorouracil (5-FU) is a promising therapeutic regimen in metastatic SCC of the head and neck [39]. Furthermore, studies are underway to investigate the efficacy of anti-angiogenic VEGF receptor inhibitors including bevacizumab in the treatment of SCC [37]. Time will reveal if these targeted therapies will become mainstay in the treatment of advanced or metastatic SCC.

As in the treatment of BCC, 5-FU and imiquimod have been trialed in the treatment of SCC in situ. 5-FU, applied twice a day for up to 9 weeks resulted in upwards of 90% clearance rate [18]. Imiquimod 5% cream applied once daily for 16 weeks can lead to a 75–80% clearance rate [18]. As previously discussed, imiquimod induces the release of a variety of cytokines and inflammatory mediators, including

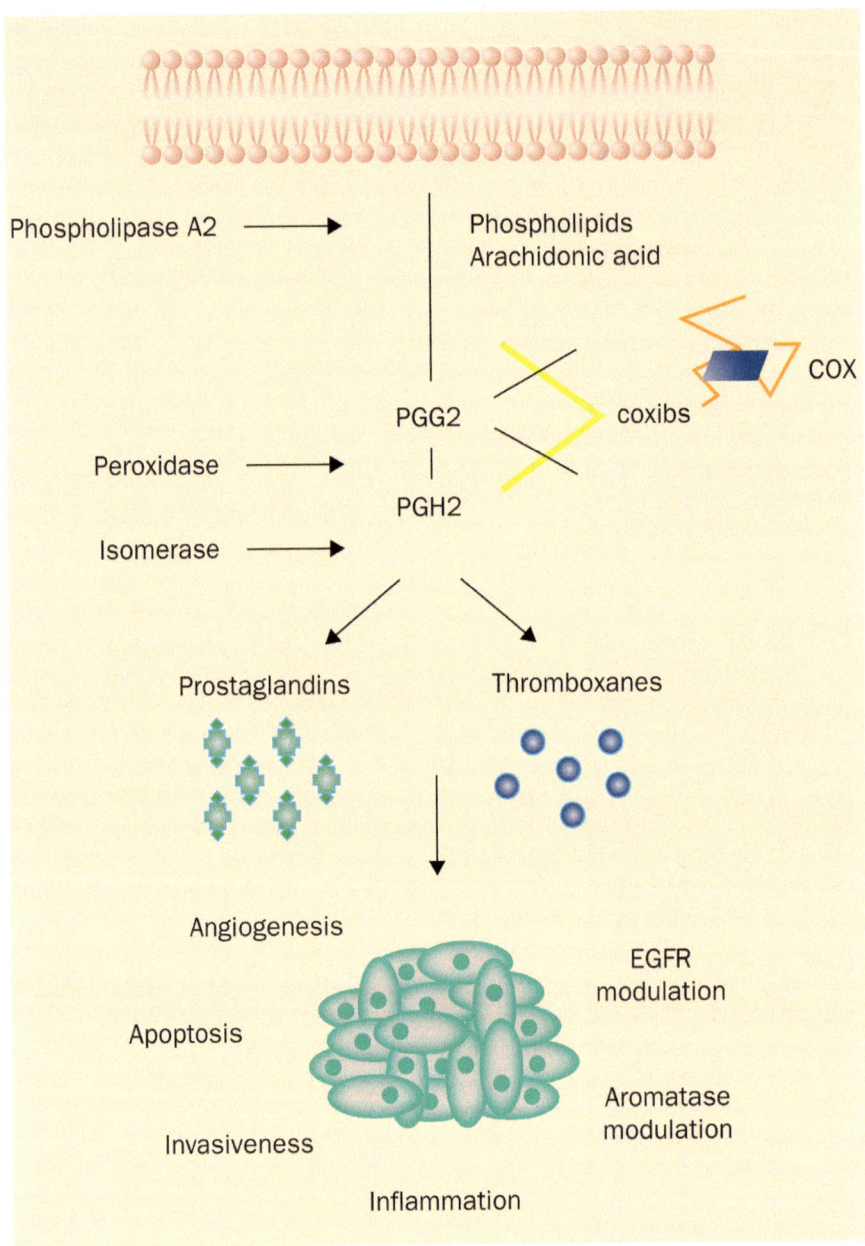

Fig. 4.4 COX catalyzes the conversion of arachidonic acid to prostaglandins, and ultimately angiogenesis and tumor progression. *COX* cyclooxygenase, *PGG2* prostaglandin G2, *PGH2* prostaglandin H2, *EGFR* epidermal growth factor receptor. (Adapted with permission from Gasparini et al. [50])

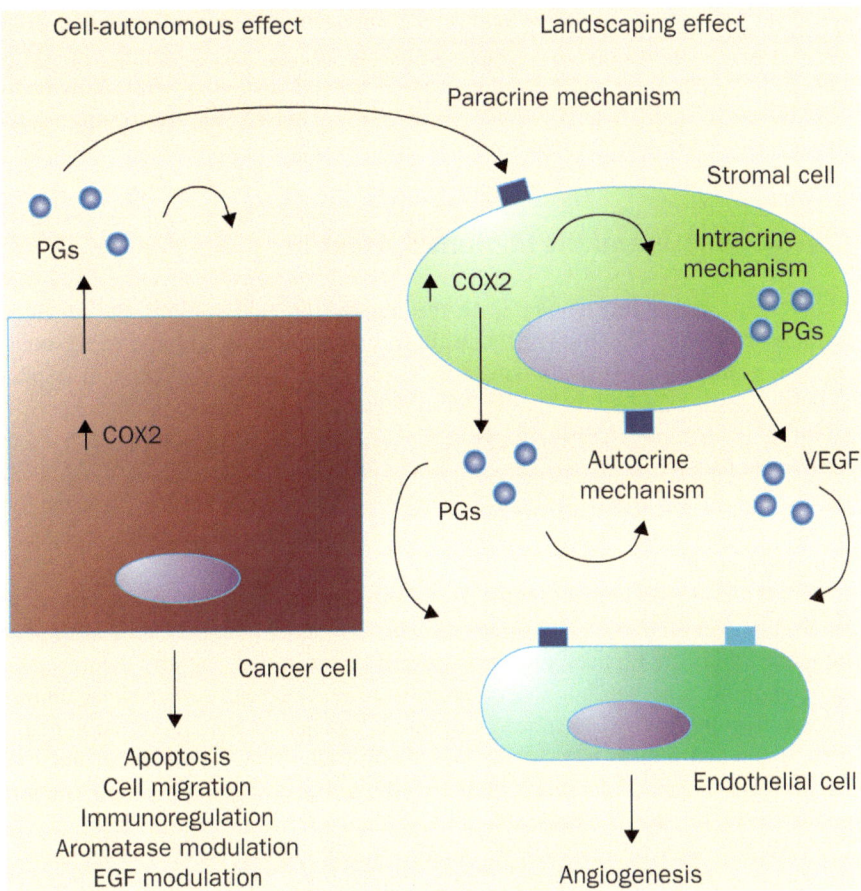

Fig. 4.5 COX-2-dependent PGs stimulate intracellular receptors (intracrine mechanism), self-prostaglandin membrane receptors (autocrine mechanism), and prostaglandin receptors on endothelial cells to promote angiogenesis. *COX-2* cyclooxygenase-2, *PGs* prostaglandins, *VEGF* vascular endothelial growth factor. (Adapted with permission from Gasparini et al. [50])

Type 1 IFNs that have potent anti-inflammatory, anti-angiogenic, and immunomodulating effects [21]. Nickoloff et al. demonstrated that human skin SCC cell lines demonstrated arrested growth when treated with IFN-α [40]. IFN-α also exerted apoptotic and immunomodulatory effects on IFN-sensitive SCC cell lines, as demonstrated by increased cellular death and decreased anti-inflammatory cytokines [21]. These preliminary findings suggest that Type 1 IFNs may play a bigger role in the nonsurgical treatment of SCC in the future.

As discussed earlier, COX-2, through the action of prostaglandin E2, is a mediator of angiogenesis, inflammation, and immunosuppression, and has been shown to be overexpressed in NMSC including SCC and BCC. Although still a debated topic, some studies seem to support that chronic non-steroidal anti-inflammatory drugs (NSAIDs) that inhibit cyclooxygenases correlate with decreased numbers of NMSC [34, 35]. In one case-control study from Australia involving 1621 individuals, NSAID use for more than two times per week for at least 1 year led to significantly lower incidences of SCC [41].

Carcinogenesis and the Immune System

Skin tumors are highly antigenic to the human immune system, and an intact immune system is essential in controlling carcinogenesis and impeding tumor growth. Immunosuppressive medications used in the treatment of organ transplant patients greatly increase the likelihood of developing UV-induced skin cancers; in addition, these tumors are more aggressive [32]. Organ transplant patients are 65 times more likely to develop SCC and 10 times more likely to develop BCC. Although these tumors are highly antigenic, iatrogenic immunosuppression impairs the immune system, allowing for unregulated development of invasive, aggressive malignancies [32].

In addition to medication-induced immunosuppression, UV light itself impairs local cutaneous immunity. In some studies, UV-radiation-naive mice who were implanted with UV-induced tumors exhibited tumor growth initially then eventual tumor regression as their immune defenses were activated and destroyed the tumors; mice who were exposed to subcarcinogenic UV-radiation prior, eventually died of their implanted tumors. These studies demonstrated that UV-radiation not only induces carcinogenic mutations in skin cells, but also impairs the host immune defense response that is responsible for the eradication of these aberrant cells [32]. UV radiation decreases the number of circulating antigen-presenting cells, impairs the function of antigen-presenting cells, stimulates the production of regulatory T cells, augments the production of the immunosuppressive cytokine IL-10, and diminishes the production of IL-12 [42–46].

Conclusion

The incidence of NMSC is rising. Although surgical excision remains the gold standard of treatment, novel systemic and topical therapeutic modalities have emerged, especially in the treatment of nonsurgical, advanced, or metastatic cases. The development of these modalities has depended on a detailed understanding and exploration of the pathogenesis of NMSC. Laboratory and clinical experiments have helped elucidate the genetic, immunologic and angiogenic factors that aid in the development of skin cancer. As a result, newer topical and systemic treatments that target these mechanisms have come to the forefront. Although much innovation has occurred, there is much more research yet to transpire. The insight into the development of skin cancer and the future of its treatment remain fruitful.

References

1. Rubin AI, Chen EH, Ratner D. Basal-cell carcinoma. N Engl J Med. 2005;353(21):2262–9.
2. Glass AG, Hoover RN. The emerging epidemic of melanoma and squamous cell skin cancer. JAMA. 1989;262(15):2097–100.
3. Rogers HW, Weinstock MA, Harris AR, Hinckley MR, Feldman SR, Fleischer AB, et al. Incidence estimate of nonmelanoma skin cancer in the united states, 2006. Arch Dermatol. 2010;146(3):283–7.
4. Diffey BL, Langtry JA. Skin cancer incidence and the ageing population. Br J Dermatol. 2005;153(3):679–80.
5. Lear JT, Smith AG. Basal cell carcinoma. Postgrad Med J. 1997;73(863):538–42.
6. Jacobs GH, Rippey JJ, Altini M. Prediction of aggressive behavior in basal cell carcinoma. Cancer. 1982;49(3):533–7.
7. Gupta AK, Daigle D, Martin G. Basal cell carcinoma. Skinmed 2014;12(1):33–38; quiz 38.
8. Martinelli E, De Palma R, Orditura M, De Vita F, Ciardiello F. Anti-epidermal growth factor receptor monoclonal antibodies in cancer therapy. Clin Exp Immunol. 2009;158(1):1–9.
9. Nagase T, Nagase M, Machida M, Fujita T. Hedgehog signalling in vascular development. Angiogenesis. 2008;11(1):71–7.
10. Lavine KJ, White AC, Park C, Smith CS, Choi K, Long F, et al. Fibroblast growth factor signals regulate a wave of hedgehog activation that is essential for coronary vascular development. Genes Dev. 2006;20(12):1651–66.
11. van Tuyl M, Groenman F, Wang J, Kuliszewski M, Liu J, Tibboel D, et al. Angiogenic factors stimulate tubular branching morphogenesis of sonic hedgehog-deficient lungs. Dev Biol. 2007;303(2):514–26.
12. Pola R, Ling LE, Aprahamian TR, Barban E, Bosch-Marce M, Curry C, et al. Postnatal recapitulation of embryonic hedgehog pathway in response to skeletal muscle ischemia. Circulation. 2003;108(4):479–85.
13. Olsen CL, Hsu PP, Glienke J, Rubanyi GM, Brooks AR. Hedgehog-interacting protein is highly expressed in endothelial cells but down-regulated during angiogenesis and in several human tumors. BMC Cancer. 2004;4:43.
14. LoRusso PM, Rudin CM, Reddy JC, Tibes R, Weiss GJ, Borad MJ, et al. Phase I trial of hedgehog pathway inhibitor vismodegib (GDC-0449) in patients with refractory, locally advanced or metastatic solid tumors. Clin Cancer Res. 2011;17(8):2502–11.
15. Muller H, Eisendle K, Gastl G, Hopfl R, Zelger B. Palliative therapy of giant basal cell carcinoma with the monoclonal anti-epidermal growth factor receptor antibody cetuximab. Br J Dermatol. 2008;158(6):1386–8.
16. Caron J, Dereure O, Kerob D, Lebbe C, Guillot B. Metastatic basal cell carcinoma: Report of two cases treated with cetuximab. Br J Dermatol. 2009;161(3):702–3.
17. Kalapurakal SJ, Malone J, Robbins KT, Buescher L, Godwin J, Rao K. Cetuximab in refractory skin cancer treatment. J Cancer. 2012;3:257–61.
18. Micali G, Lacarrubba F, Nasca MR, Ferraro S, Schwartz RA. Topical pharmacotherapy for skin cancer: Part II. clinical applications. J Am Acad Dermatol 2014;70(6):979e.1–12; quiz 9912.
19. Dubas LE, Ingraffea A. Nonmelanoma skin cancer. Facial Plast Surg Clin North Am. 2013;21(1):43–53.
20. Gaspari A, Tyring SK, Rosen T. Beyond a decade of 5% imiquimod topical therapy. J Drugs Dermatol. 2009;8(5):467–74.
21. Ismail A, Yusuf N. Type I interferons: key players in normal skin and select cutaneous malignancies. Dermatol Res Pract. 2014;2014:847545.
22. Kim KH, Yavel RM, Gross VL, Brody N. Intralesional interferon alpha-2b in the treatment of basal cell carcinoma and squamous cell carcinoma: Revisited. Dermatol Surg. 2004;30(1):116–20.

23. Stout AJ, Gresser I, Thompson WD. Inhibition of wound healing in mice by local interferon alpha/beta injection. Int J Exp Pathol. 1993;74(1):79–85.
24. McCarty MF, Bielenberg D, Donawho C, Bucana CD, Fidler IJ. Evidence for the causal role of endogenous interferon-alpha/beta in the regulation of angiogenesis, tumorigenicity, and metastasis of cutaneous neoplasms. Clin Exp Metastasis. 2002;19(7):609–15.
25. Niederwieser D, Aubock J, Troppmair J, Herold M, Schuler G, Boeck G, et al. IFN-mediated induction of MHC antigen expression on human keratinocytes and its influence on in vitro alloimmune responses. J Immunol. 1988;140(8):2556–64.
26. Urosevic M, Oberholzer PA, Maier T, Hafner J, Laine E, Slade H, et al. Imiquimod treatment induces expression of opioid growth factor receptor: a novel tumor antigen induced by interferon-alpha? Clin Cancer Res. 2004;10(15):4959–70.
27. Buechner SA, Wernli M, Harr T, Hahn S, Itin P, Erb P. Regression of basal cell carcinoma by intralesional interferon-alpha treatment is mediated by CD95 (apo-1/Fas)-CD95 ligand-induced suicide. J Clin Invest. 1997;100(11):2691–6.
28. Buechner SA. Intralesional interferon alfa-2b in the treatment of basal cell carcinoma. immunohistochemical study on cellular immune reaction leading to tumor regression. J Am Acad Dermatol. 1991;24(5 Pt 1):731–4.
29. Mozzanica N, Cattaneo A, Boneschi V, Brambilla L, Melotti E, Finzi AF. Immunohistological evaluation of basal cell carcinoma immunoinfiltrate during intralesional treatment with alpha 2-interferon. Arch Dermatol Res. 1990;282(5):311–7.
30. Findlay GM. Ultra-violet light and skin cancer. CA Cancer J Clin. 1979;29(3):169–71.
31. Brash DE, Rudolph JA, Simon JA, Lin A, McKenna GJ, Baden HP, et al. A role for sunlight in skin cancer: UV-induced p53 mutations in squamous cell carcinoma. Proc Natl Acad Sci U S A. 1991;88(22):10124–8.
32. Elmets CA, Athar M. Milestones in photocarcinogenesis. J Invest Dermatol. 2013;133(E1):E13–7.
33. An KP, Athar M, Tang X, Katiyar SK, Russo J, Beech J, et al. Cyclooxygenase-2 expression in murine and human nonmelanoma skin cancers: Implications for therapeutic approaches. Photochem Photobiol. 2002;76(1):73–80.
34. Elmets CA, Ledet JJ, Athar M. Cyclooxygenases: mediators of UV-induced skin cancer and potential targets for prevention. J Invest Dermatol. 2014;134(10):2497–502.
35. Elmets CA, Viner JL, Pentland AP, Cantrell W, Lin HY, Bailey H, et al. Chemoprevention of nonmelanoma skin cancer with celecoxib: a randomized, double-blind, placebo-controlled trial. J Natl Cancer Inst. 2010;102(24):1835–44.
36. Boeckx C, Baay M, Wouters A, Specenier P, Vermorken JB, Peeters M, et al. Anti-epidermal growth factor receptor therapy in head and neck squamous cell carcinoma: focus on potential molecular mechanisms of drug resistance. Oncologist. 2013;18(7):850–64.
37. O'Bryan KW, Ratner D. The role of targeted molecular inhibitors in the management of advanced nonmelanoma skin cancer. Semin Cutan Med Surg. 2011;30(1):57–61.
38. Bonner JA, Harari PM, Giralt J, Cohen RB, Jones CU, Sur RK, et al. Radiotherapy plus cetuximab for locoregionally advanced head and neck cancer: 5-year survival data from a phase 3 randomised trial, and relation between cetuximab-induced rash and survival. Lancet Oncol. 2010;11(1):21–8.
39. Vermorken JB, Mesia R, Rivera F, Remenar E, Kawecki A, Rottey S, et al. Platinum-based chemotherapy plus cetuximab in head and neck cancer. N Engl J Med. 2008;359(11):1116–27.
40. Nickoloff BJ, Basham TY, Merigan TC, Morhenn VB. Immunomodulatory and antiproliferative effect of recombinant alpha, beta, and gamma interferons on cultured human malignant squamous cell lines, SCL-1 and SW-1271. J Invest Dermatol. 1985;84(6):487–90.
41. Butler GJ, Neale R, Green AC, Pandeya N, Whiteman DC. Nonsteroidal anti-inflammatory drugs and the risk of actinic keratoses and squamous cell cancers of the skin. J Am Acad Dermatol. 2005;53(6):966–72.

42. Toews GB, Bergstresser PR, Streilein JW. Epidermal langerhans cell density determines whether contact hypersensitivity or unresponsiveness follows skin painting with DNFB. J Immunol. 1980;124(1):445–53.
43. Elmets CA, Bergstresser PR, Tigelaar RE, Wood PJ, Streilein JW. Analysis of the mechanism of unresponsiveness produced by haptens painted on skin exposed to low dose ultraviolet radiation. J Exp Med. 1983;158(3):781–94.
44. Schwarz A, Grabbe S, Aragane Y, Sandkuhl K, Riemann H, Luger TA, et al. Interleukin-12 prevents ultraviolet B-induced local immunosuppression and overcomes UVB-induced tolerance. J Invest Dermatol. 1996;106(6):1187–91.
45. Shreedhar V, Giese T, Sung VW, Ullrich SE. A cytokine cascade including prostaglandin E2, IL-4, and IL-10 is responsible for UV-induced systemic immune suppression. J Immunol. 1998;160(8):3783–9.
46. Loser K, Apelt J, Voskort M, Mohaupt M, Balkow S, Schwarz T, et al. IL-10 controls ultraviolet-induced carcinogenesis in mice. J Immunol. 2007;179(1):365–71.
47. Madan V, Lear JT, Szeimies RM. Non-melanoma skin cancer. Lancet. 2010;375(9715):673–85.
48. Epstein EH. Basal cell carcinomas: attack of the hedgehog. Nat Rev Cancer. 2008;8(10):743–54.
49. Ulevitch RJ. Therapeutics targeting the innate immune system. Nat Rev Immunol. 2004;4(7):512–20.
50. Gasparini G, Longo R, Sarmiento R, Morabito A. Inhibitors of cyclo-oxygenase 2: a new class of anticancer agents? Lancet Oncol. 2003;4(10):605–15.

Melanoma

5

Julide Tok Celebi

Abbreviations and Glossary of Terms

ANG	Angiopoietin; growth factor
bFGF	basic fibroblast growth factor or fibroblast growth factor 2; growth factor
BRAF	v-raf murine sarcoma viral oncogene homolog B; the most commonly mutated oncogene in melanoma
CTLA-4	Cytotoxic T-lymphocyte-associated protein 4; receptor; inhibitor for T cell activation
FGF	Fibroblast growth factor; growth factor
FGFR	Fibroblast growth factor receptor; receptor
FLT-3	Fms-like tyrosine kinase 3; receptor
FZD	Frizzled class receptor; receptor
IGF	Insulin growth factor; growth factor
KIT	v-Kit Hardy-Zuckerman 4 feline sarcoma viral oncogene homolog; receptor
MEK	Mitogen-activated protein kinase kinase 1; signaling molecule critical for transducing signals in the RAS-RAF-MEK-ERK (MAPK; mitogen-activated protein kinase) pathway
PDGF	Platelet-derived growth factor; growth factor
PDGFR	Platelet-derived growth factor receptor; receptor
PD1	Programmed cell death 1; receptor, inhibits T cell activation and turn off cytotoxic T cells

J.T. Celebi, MD
Department of Dermatology, Department of Pathology, Icahn School of Medicine at Mount Sinai, New York, NY, USA
e-mail: julide.celebi@mountsinai.org

© Springer-Verlag London Ltd. 2017
J.L. Arbiser (ed.), *Angiogenesis-Based Dermatology*,
DOI 10.1007/978-1-4471-7314-4_5

PD-L1   Programmed cell death 1 ligand; ligand; inhibits T cell activation and
         turn off cytotoxic T cells
VEGF   Vascular endothelial growth factor; growth factor
VEGFR   Vascular endothelial growth factor receptor; receptor
WNT   Wingless-type MMTV integration site family; growth factor

Introduction

Melanoma is potentially a fatal malignancy with more than 76,250 estimated new cases of invasive melanoma in the United States annually resulting in over 9180 deaths [1]. It is the fifth and sixth most common cancer in men and women, respectively [1]. Early disease is typically cured with surgery however advanced disease has a poor prognosis.

Prior to the successful use of targeted therapies and immune modulators, the overall survival of a patient with widespread melanoma was approximately 3–6 months. The breakthrough started when a BRAF inhibitor [2] and immune checkpoint blockade CTLA-4 antibody [3], showed significant clinical responses in patients with late-stage disease. Due to recent advances in the therapeutic arena over the past 4 years, overall survival for patients with advanced metastatic melanoma has extended beyond 15–20 months and thus it is no longer limited to 3–6 months.

An exciting therapeutic momentum began with the BRAF inhibitor, vemurafenib, and the CTLA-4 antibody, ipilimumab, receiving their US Food and Drug Administration (FDA) approvals for the treatment of late-stage melanoma in 2011. Although various genetic aberrations have been described, BRAF is the most frequently mutated oncogene in melanoma, resulting in activation of the RAS-RAF-MEK-ERK signaling pathway [4]. Pharmacological inhibition of this signaling cascade is successful in tumor reduction. BRAF inhibitors show significant clinical efficacy in BRAF-mutant melanomas with over 50% of response and improve overall survival up to 16 months [2]. MEK inhibitors in combination with BRAF inhibition improve survival even beyond [5, 6]. However, patients eventually relapse due to acquisition of resistance [7, 8]. Immunologic-based treatments targeting CTLA-4, PD1, or PDL1 inhibit negative T cell responses that lead to T cell activation and tumor cell killing. Recent studies show significant clinical activity in a subset of patients with durable responses [9, 10]. Some patients receiving ipilimumab achieve long-term responses up to 4.5 years. However, not all patients respond to this treatment approach and some experience severe immune-related adverse effects [10]. As new therapeutic targets are being identified, new drugs being developed, and new combinatorial regimens are being tested, alternative approaches such as targeting the angiogenesis program are of significant interest in the field.

Angiogenesis in Melanoma: The Science

Tumor Angiogenesis

Angiogenesis is defined as new vessel growth that is essential for local tumor growth by providing oxygen and nutrients for tumor cells as well as for metastatic spread by providing channels for tumor cell dissemination to other sites (Fig. 5.1) [11]. Angiogenic activity depends on the balance of positive and negative modulators that tightly regulate the behavior of the vascular endothelium. In healthy skin tissue, the vasculature remains quiescent due to dominance of negative regulators of angiogenesis (anti-angiogenic factors). During tumor development, the balance shifts in favor of pro-angiogenic factors that contribute to the process of neo-vascularization and tumor angiogenesis. During this process, there is downregulation of negative regulators and an increase in positive regulators that are mainly released by neoplastic cells and immune cells that ultimately lead to the growth of new blood vessels. Tumor angiogenesis, however, is not limited to an increase in blood vessel density, but also represents various structural and functional abnormalities of the vessels that are usually associated with increased permeability allowing trafficking of tumor cells into the circulation.

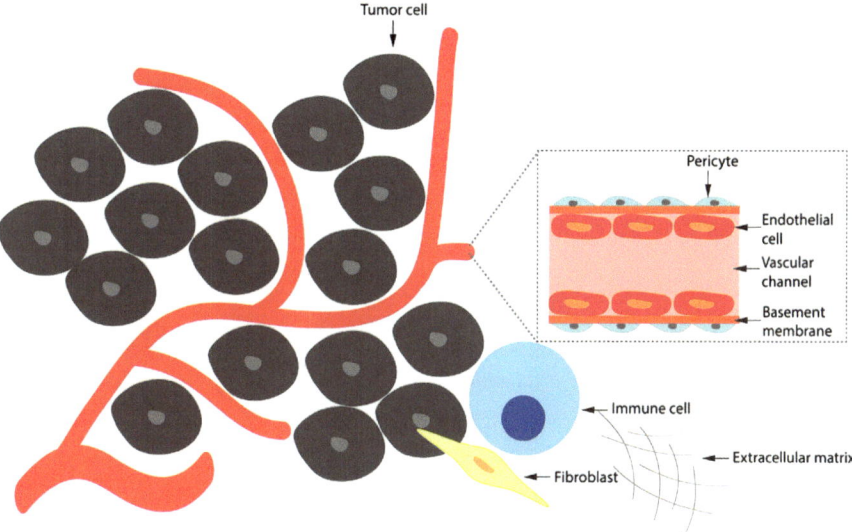

Fig. 5.1 Tumor Angiogenesis. Blood vessels, tumor cells, and the cells of the tumor microenvironment are schematically depicted. Enlarged image (*right panel*) shows the cross section of a blood vessel.

Mechanisms of Tumor Angiogenesis in Melanoma

There are several modes of tumor vascularization. For many years, the process of tumor vascularization was thought to mainly involve sprouting of new blood vessels from pre-existing vasculature (sprouting angiogenesis). However, in recent years, additional mechanisms have been recognized, such as vascular co-option, intussusceptive angiogenesis, mosaic vessels, bone marrow-derived vasculogenesis, and vasculogenic mimicry [12–15].

Sprouting Angiogenesis – the growth of new capillary vessels from pre-existing ones - has been the most studied mechanism of neo-vascularization over the years [11, 12, 16] (Fig. 5.2). It involves endothelial cell proliferation, migration, and tube (vascular channel) formation. There are three sequential steps; quiescence, activation, and resolution. Every step involves well-coordinated molecular signaling. Mechanistically, it begins with basement membrane degradation of the endothelium and disruption of this monolayer [12]. When a quiescent vessel senses an angiogenic signal (e.g. growth factors such as VEGF, ANG-2, FGFs, and cytokines) released by the tumor cell, pericytes first detach from the vessel wall and liberate themselves from the basement membrane by proteolytic degradation (mediated by matrix metalloproteinases). Endothelial cells loosen their junctions, the nascent vessel dilates, plasma proteins and others extravasate to form an angio-competent milieu. To form a perfused tube (a new vessel) one endothelial cell, known as the

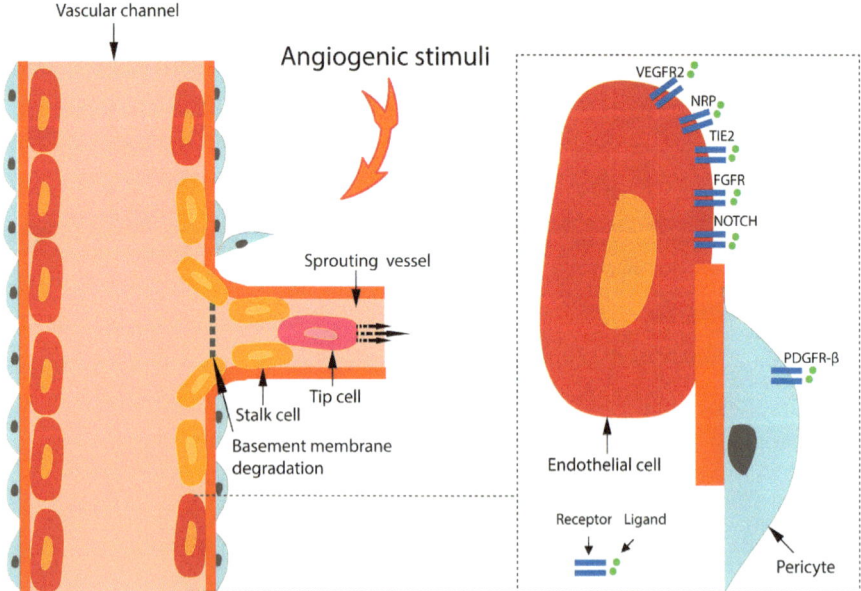

Fig. 5.2 Sprouting Angiogenesis. The process of neo-vascularization in sprouting angiogenesis is shown. Enlarged image (*right panel*) shows the key ligand-receptor interactions on the surface of the endothelial cells.

'tip cell', becomes selected to lead the tip. VEGFRs, neuropilins, and the NOTCH receptors are critical for this step. The neighbors of the tip cell, known as the 'stalk cells', divide and establish the lumen followed by initiation of blood flow, deposition of basement membrane, and pericyte coverage. During maturation, stalk cells transform into phalanx cells. The end result of this process is a new perfused vascular channel from a pre-existing one.

Tumor Microenvironment During Angiogenesis

Tumor angiogenesis was first thought to be fueled by neoplastic cells, however emerging evidence suggests that the tumor microenvironment and the immune cell subsets are as important for regulating this process (Table 5.1) [17, 18]. There appears to be a complex but well orchestrated interplay between the neoplastic cells, immune cells, and the vascular endothelium [12, 19]. Tumor cells disrupt normal tissue homeostasis by altering its gene expression to secrete molecules (e.g. growth factors and cytokines) and cellular components to recruit other cell types. Early in the course of tumor growth, hypoxia leads to activation of hypoxia-inducible factor that follows a rapid increase in blood vessel formation. Cells of the tumor microenvironment are heterogeneous in origin, and can be derived from the stroma, blood vessels, or the bone marrow [16].

Angiogenic Factors in Melanoma

A number of pro-angiogenic growth factors essential for melanoma growth and metastasis have been characterized. They function via the classic ligand-receptor interaction; the growth factor released from the tumor cell or other cells within the

Table 5.1 Tumor microenvironment in angiogenesis

Tumor microenvironment	Major constituents
1. Cells (a) Tumor cells (b) Immune cells (c) Pericytes	Melanoma cells Monocytes, macrophages, myeloid derived suppressor cells, dendritic cells, natural killer cells, neutrophils, mast cells, eosinophils, T and B cells, plasma cells
2. Stroma (a) Extracellular matrix (b) Fibroblasts (c) Myofibroblasts (d) Endothelial cells	Collagen, fibronectin, laminin, proteoglycan
3. Soluble factors (a) Pro-angiogenic (b) Anti-angiogenic (c) Proteases	VEGFs, PDGFs, Ang-1/2, PROK-1/2, FGFs, EGF, IGF, HGF, PlGF Thrombospodin-1, angiostatin, endostatin Matrix metalloproteinases, u-PA, elastase

microenvironment binds to its specific receptor expressed on the endothelial cell and enhances signaling leading to endothelial cell proliferation and migration (Fig. 5.2). While these growth factors are typically secreted or released by the tumor cell, some are let-off by the stromal cells, bone marrow derived progenitor cells, and/or inflammatory cells. Some of the key pro-angiogenic growth factors, their receptors, and contribution to the angiogenesis program in melanoma are reviewed.

The VEGF (Vascular Endothelial Growth Factor) Family VEGF family is a large group of growth factors including VEGF-A, -B, -C, -D, -E, and placental growth factor-1 and -2 (PIGF-1 and -2) [20–22]. VEGF-A (also referred as VEGF) is the main component that regulates angiogenesis in health and disease [23]. VEGFR-2 is the predominant receptor tyrosine kinase that mediates VEGF signaling in endothelial cells and that drives VEGF-mediated angiogenesis. VEGFs bind to three structurally similar tyrosine kinase receptors VEGFR-1 (Flt-1), VEGFR-2 (Flk-1, KDR) and VEGFR-3 (Flt-4) to stimulate blood vessel proliferation and angiogenesis [21]. VEGFR-1 and -2 are expressed almost exclusively on endothelial cells, while VEGFR-3 is necessary for blood vasculature during early embryogenesis, but later becomes a key regulator of lymphangiogenesis, the formation of new lymphatic vessels. While VEGFR-1 and -2 are involved in angiogenesis by VEGF-A isoform, VEGFR-3 is involved in lymphangiogenesis by VEGF-C and -D. Neuropilin-1 and -2 are members of the VEGF family that function as co-receptors to enhance binding to VEGFR-2, but also can signal independently.

VEGF is upregulated in melanoma, but is not expressed in normal melanocytes [24]. Increased expression of VEGF and VEGFRs in primary cutaneous melanoma as well as increased microvascular density strongly correlates with disease progression [25–27]. Serum VEGF levels are increased in melanoma patients compared with healthy controls [28].

The PDGF (Platelet-derived Growth Factor) Family PDGF is a family of five growth factors (PDGF-AA, -AB, -BB, -CC, and -DD) that exert their biological effects through tyrosine kinase receptors, PDGFR-α and -β [21, 22]. The PDGF isoforms differ in their receptor specificity. The -A and -C chains bind only to PDGFR-α, and the -D chain binds only to PDGFR-β, whereas the -B chain binds to both. PDGFs together with angiopoietins and TGF-β have critical roles in endothelial cell-pericyte interaction [29]. During angiogenesis, endothelial cells produce PDGF-BB that stimulates PDGFR-β-expressing pericytes, and result in proliferation and migration of pericytes. Pericytes provide coverage of the vessel wall to stabilize the channels. Either PDGFR inhibition or pericyte deficiency leads to vessel leakage, tortuosity, and immature vessel formation. In the context of tumor angiogenesis, pericyte coverage of the vessel walls appears to be protective against metastasis as endothelial channels lined with pericytes limit tumor cell intravasation as opposed to those that are loosely assembled and leaky [30].

Melanomas show enhanced expression of PDGF-AA, −BB, and PDGFR-α [31]. In highly metastatic melanoma cell lines, expression of PDGFR-α is significantly elevated as compared to PDGFR-β.

The FGF (Fibroblast Growth Factor) Superfamily FGFs activate receptors (FGFR1-4) on endothelial cells or indirectly stimulate angiogenesis by inducing the release of angiogenic factors from other cell types [12]. Low levels of FGF are required for the maintenance of vascular integrity. Aberrant FGF signaling promotes tumor angiogenesis.

bFGF (basic FGF or FGF-2) has been well studied in melanocytic tumors. It is expressed in melanoma cells but not in normal melanocytes [32]. Targeting bFGF in melanoma cells decrease tumor growth in vitro and in vivo [33].

ANG-TIE Signaling The ANG (Angiopoietin) family is composed of at least three ligands (ANG-1, -2, and -4) and two tyrosine kinase receptors, TIE-1 and TIE-2. ANG-1 functions as a TIE-2 agonist, stimulates mural coverage and vessel tightness, and is critical for maintenance of endothelial cell quiescence. Whereas ANG-2 when stimulated by angiogenic factors antagonizes the ANG-1 and TIE-2 signaling to enhance mural cell detachment, vascular permeability, and endothelial cell sprouting. Thus, ANG-1/TIE-2 and ANG-2 function in a reciprocal manner as anti- or pro-angiogenic, respectively.

Elevated serum levels of ANG-2 are reported in patients with melanoma compared with healthy individuals [34]. Circulating levels of ANG-2 correlates with stage of disease and overall survival.

NOTCH Signaling There are three ligands (Delta-like 4, Jagged-1 and -2) and four NOTCH receptors (NOTCH 1–4) [35]. DLL4 and NOTCH signaling is critical for generating perfused vessels, tip cell selection, stalk cell proliferation [35]. The activity of this signaling is low during vessel quiescence. In tumor angiogenesis, inhibition of Delta-like 4/NOTCH signaling induces more but hypoperfused vessels, resulting in growth inhibition.

WNT Signaling Endothelial cells express various types of WNT ligand and their frizzled (FZD) receptors, of which several stimulate endothelial cell proliferation [36]. NOTCH and WNT activate each other in a reciprocal-feedback system [36]. WNT and NOTCH result in a similar phenotype in endothelial cells, characterized by branching defects, loss of venous identity and aberrant vascular modeling.

Angiogenesis in Melanoma: The Therapeutic Implications

Targeting VEGF

The concept of anti-angiogenesis therapy was coined by Folkman and colleagues in 1971 based on the observation that tumors do not grow beyond a minimal size of 1–2 mm^3 without new vessel formation and therefore inhibiting angiogenesis could prevent tumor progression [37]. VEGF was discovered as the primary mediator of tumor angiogenesis soon followed by generation of monoclonal antibody against this growth factor and FDA approval in 2004 [38]. A plethora of pre-clinical and clinical studies on VEGF and its inhibition including in melanoma concluded its lack of effectiveness as a single agent [38]. However, combining it with other drugs have shown clinical benefit, and thus it is approved and used only in combination with other drugs in several solid tumors [12]. Many patients are refractory or acquire resistance to VEGF inhibitors, and biomarkers to identify responders are lacking [39].

In melanoma, its combinatorial partner(s) are vigorously being sought, immune checkpoint blockade (e.g. anti-CTLA-4, anti-PD1, anti-PDL1) currently receiving immediate attention. It is likely that in the near future key drivers of angiogenesis beyond VEGF will be identified as well as bypass mechanisms when a major endothelial growth factor such as VEGF is inhibited along with a search for immune modulating and other combinatorial agents that act in synergy, thus leading to effective angiogenesis-based therapeutics. Readers can view the ongoing clinical trials targeting VEGF or others in melanoma via www.clinicaltrials.gov.

Bevacizumab (Table 5.2) This is a recombinant humanized monoclonal antibody that neutralizes VEGF isoforms [40]. Although there are many drugs that inhibit VEGF and its signaling (e.g. sorafenib, sunitinib), bevacizumab is the most commonly studied and used agent to date and considered as a prototype for anti-angiogenesis based treatments due to its selectivity. Bevacizumab combined with other neoplastic agents (e.g. interferon-alpha, chemotherapy) has been approved for the treatment of advanced non-small cell lung cancer, breast cancer, colorectal cancer, glioblastoma multiforme, and renal cell carcinoma [12]. It is also licensed for the intravitreal treatment of choroidal neovascularization secondary to age-related macular degeneration [41].

Clinical trials in melanoma concluded that Bevacizumab has little activity as a single agent for the treatment of advanced melanoma [42]. However combining VEGF inhibitors with other agents may be of interest. In some solid cancers, even though bevacizumab as monotherapy was ineffective combining with interferon or chemotherapy, lead to marked clinical improvement and is currently approved for the treatment of these tumors (e.g. colorectal cancer, renal cell carcinoma, non-small cell lung cancer, breast cancer, ovarian cancer, and glioblastoma multiforme) [43].

Table 5.2 Bevacizumab in the treatment of cancer

Bevacizumab as single agent	Ineffective

Bevacizumab in combination [interferon or chemotherapy]	Approved[a] for the treatment of
	  Metastatic colorectal cancer
	  Metastatic non-small cell lung cancer
	  Metastatic renal cell cancer
	  Recurrent glioblastoma multiforme

For reference, see http://www.clinicaltrials.gov
This summary is limited to current knowledge; many clinical trials are ongoing
[a]Approved by the FDA

This drug has been found to initially reduce tumor perfusion, vascular volume, and microvascular density, findings referred to as 'vascular normalization' [44]. This phenomenon has been proposed as a plausible explanation for the improved activity of radiotherapy and cytotoxic agents given in combination with bevacizumab, as tumor normalization improves tissue oxygen levels and drug delivery. However, unlike other cancers, the search for interferon or a chemotherapeutic agent in combination with bevacizumab with improved activity for melanoma has not yet been successful. It has been tested in combination with low dose interferon alpha-2a (plus dacarbazine) [45], high-dose interferon alpha-2b [46], or several chemotherapeutic agents in metastatic melanoma [42], but did not show significant clinical responses. Adverse effects included neutropenia, peripheral neuropathy, arterial thromboembolic events and hypertension [42].

One of the largest initial trials was the BEAM study with 214 patients investigating bevacizumab (in combination with carboplatin and paclitaxel). In this randomized phase 2 study there was no improvement in progression-free survival. At 17-month follow-up, bevacizumab prolonged the median overall survival (12.3 versus 8.6 months), with a non-significant 21% reduction in the hazard of death [42]. Bevacizumab and fotemustine showed an overall survival of 20 months in 20 patients [47]. A phase II trial combining bevacizumab and high-dose interferon alpha-2b in advanced melanoma that accrued 25 patients showed a median overall survival of 17 months [46]. In a phase II trial combining bevacizumab and temsirolimus (CTEP 7190/Mel47) for unresectable stage III/IV melanoma, three patients showed partial response (17.7%), 9 patients stable disease at 8 weeks, and 4 patients had progressive disease [48]. Temozolomide and bevacizumab in 62 patients revealed overall survival of 9.6 months (SAKK 50/07) [49]. In another phase II trial (N0775), temozolomide and bevacizumab or nab-paclitaxel, carboplatin and bevacizumab in patients with unresectable stage IV melanoma were evaluated in 93 patients and showed median overall survival of 12.3 months and 13.9 months, respectively [50].

In preclinical studies VEGF has been associated with anti-tumor responses, including suppression of dendritic-cell maturation, proliferation of regulatory T cells, inhibition of T-cell responses, and accumulation of myeloid-derived suppressor cells [51–55]. Thus, combining VEGF inhibition with immune checkpoint blockers (e.g. anti-CTLA-4) plus given the success of ipilimumab in the clinical setting was the next logical step. In a recent study bevacizumab and ipilimumab combination resulted in partial responses in 8 patients and stable disease 22 patients in a phase I trial of 46 patients [56]. Disease control rate in this study was 67.4% and median survival was 25.1 months. In an earlier study, ipilimumab, when compared with gp100 peptide vaccine improved the median overall survival from 6.4 to 10.1 months [3]. Therefore, the study combining ipilimumab with bevacizumab suggests worthy of future pursuit towards this combination. Notably, inflammatory toxicities were generally higher with the combination therapy than ipilimumab alone but were manageable [56].

Bevacizumab in the Adjuvant Setting There is a need to improve adjuvant treatment for patients who have melanoma and are at high risk of disease recurrence after surgery. Adjuvant use of bevacizumab in this context was examined (AVAST-M study). A large phase III open-label multicenter clinical trial published in 2014 randomized 1343 patients with resected cutaneous melanoma at high risk for recurrence (stage IIB, IIC, and III) to either bevacizumab group (n = 671) or the observation group (n = 672). One hundred thirty four (96%) patients in the bevacizumab died of melanoma versus 139 (95%) in the observation group. There was no significance in overall survival between the groups at a median of 51 weeks of treatment. At this point, one can conclude that adjuvant use of bevacizumab in melanoma is not beneficial. This finding is not surprising, as the adjuvant use of this drug has not improved survival in patients with any other tumor type to date [57]. Nevertheless, longer follow up to meet the 5-year survival end point will determine the final beneficial effects and risks of this drug in melanoma [58].

Bevacizumab in Uveal Melanoma Uveal melanoma is a subtype of melanoma that arises from melanocytes of the uveal tract [59]. Apart from its difference from cutaneous melanoma in its anatomic location, developmental pathways, clinical characteristics, genetic aberrations, and prognosis, it metastasizes through the hematogenous route, typically to the liver, and is an angiogenic tumor [59]. Levels of VEGF are significantly elevated in patients with metastatic disease compared to patients without metastases [60]. IGF-1 has been shown to stimulate secretion of VEGF in retinal pigment epithelial cells and IGF-1 signaling may also stimulate tumor angiogenesis in uveal melanoma liver metastases [61].

Anti-angiogenesis therapy has not yet been used for the standard treatment of primary uveal melanoma or related metastatic diseases, although the intravitreal application of bevacizumab has been successfully applied in non-oncologic neovascularization diseases such as macular degeneration and proliferative diabetic retinopathy. There has been extensive research into the effect of anti-angiogenic agents such as bevacizumab on uveal melanoma cells in vitro and in animal models [61, 62]. Yang et al. studied the effect of bevacizumab on the growth and number of hepatic micrometastases in a mouse model of ocular melanoma: systemic bevacizumab suppressed primary ocular melanoma growth and the formation of hepatic micrometastases in a dose-dependent manner. In addition, bevacizumab reduced the level of VEGF in the culture media of two human uveal melanoma cell lines [61]. Clinical trials using intravitreal bevacizumab in uveal melanoma are either on going or have recently been completed.

Other VEGF Inhibitors

Ranibizumab is a recombinant humanized monoclonal antibody fragment that specifically binds VEGF-A. It is currently only approved for the intravitreal treatment of macular degeneration. Aflibercept (VEGF Trap) is a fusion protein combining the Fc portion of human IgG1 with the principal extracellular ligand-binding domains of human VEGFR1 and VEGFR2. It acts as a high-affinity soluble trap to the VEGF receptor and is thus a potent angiogenesis inhibitor [63].

Additionally, there are VEGFR tyrosine kinase inhibitors. These *small* molecules target the intracellular tyrosine kinase domain of multiple receptors (termed *multi-tyrosine kinase inhibitors*), most notably the VEGFR. They act by reversibly attaching to the ATP binding site, blocking the enzymatic action of the kinases and ultimately inhibiting the pathologically increased signal transduction in the malignant cell. One such drug sorafenib is an oral multi-kinase inhibitor that that is licensed for the treatment of renal cell carcinoma and hepatocellular carcinoma [64]. Sorafenib can inhibit several serine-threonine and receptor kinases including RAF, VEGFR-2 and VEGFR-3, PDGFR-β, Fms-like tyrosine kinase 3 (FLT-3) and c-Kit protein (KIT) [65]. Sunitinib is another small molecule approved for the treatment of advanced and/or metastatic renal cell carcinoma [64] and for unresectable and/or metastatic malignant gastrointestinal stromal tumor after unsuccessful imatinib therapy [66]. This multikinase inhibitor selectively targets PDGFR-α and -β, VEGFR-1, −2 and −3, KIT, FLT-3 and the RET receptor [67]. Several new multi-kinase inhibitors have recently appeared in the market and have been approved for the treatment of several malignancies. These include pazopanib, cediranib, vandetanib, and axitinib [68]. These drugs affect several receptors including the VEGFR-1, 2, and 3.

Acknowledgements Julide Celebi is funded by the National Institutes of Health/National Cancer Institute (CA138678, CA158557, CA177940), the Melanoma Research Foundation, and a Pilot Program Project from the Icahn School of Medicine at Mount Sinai. We apologize to authors whose work could not be cited due to space limitations.

References

1. Siegel R, Naishadham D, Jemal A. Cancer statistics, 2013. CA Cancer J Clin. 2013;63(1):11–30.
2. Sosman JA, Kim KB, Schuchter L, Gonzalez R, Pavlick AC, Weber JS, et al. Survival in BRAF V600-mutant advanced melanoma treated with vemurafenib. N Engl J Med. 2012;366(8):707–14.
3. Hodi FS, O'Day SJ, McDermott DF, Weber RW, Sosman JA, Haanen JB, et al. Improved survival with ipilimumab in patients with metastatic melanoma. N Engl J Med. 2010;363(8):711–23.
4. Davies H, Bignell GR, Cox C, Stephens P, Edkins S, Clegg S, et al. Mutations of the BRAF gene in human cancer. Nature. 2002;417(6892):949–54.
5. Menzies AM, Long GV. Dabrafenib and trametinib, alone and in combination for BRAF-mutant metastatic melanoma. Clin Cancer Res Off J Am Assoc Cancer Res. 2014;20(8):2035–43.
6. Larkin J, Ascierto PA, Dreno B, Atkinson V, Liszkay G, Maio M, et al. Combined vemurafenib and cobimetinib in BRAF-mutated melanoma. N Engl J Med. 2014;371(20):1867–76.
7. Bucheit AD, Davies MA. Emerging insights into resistance to BRAF inhibitors in melanoma. Biochem Pharmacol. 2014;87(3):381–9.
8. Lito P, Rosen N, Solit DB. Tumor adaptation and resistance to RAF inhibitors. Nat Med. 2013;19(11):1401–9.
9. Wolchok JD, Kluger H, Callahan MK, Postow MA, Rizvi NA, Lesokhin AM, et al. Nivolumab plus ipilimumab in advanced melanoma. N Engl J Med. 2013;369(2):122–33.

10. Naidoo J, Page DB, Wolchok JD. Immune modulation for cancer therapy. Br J Cancer. 2014;111(12):2214–9.
11. Welti J, Loges S, Dimmeler S, Carmeliet P. Recent molecular discoveries in angiogenesis and antiangiogenic therapies in cancer. J Clin Invest. 2013;123(8):3190–200.
12. Carmeliet P, Jain RK. Molecular mechanisms and clinical applications of angiogenesis. Nature. 2011;473(7347):298–307.
13. Wang R, Chadalavada K, Wilshire J, Kowalik U, Hovinga KE, Geber A, et al. Glioblastoma stem-like cells give rise to tumour endothelium. Nature. 2010;468(7325):829–33.
14. Pastushenko I, Vermeulen PB, Van den Eynden GG, Rutten A, Carapeto FJ, Dirix LY, et al. Mechanisms of tumour vascularization in cutaneous malignant melanoma: clinical implications. Br J Dermatol. 2014;171(2):220–33.
15. Hendrix MJ, Seftor EA, Hess AR, Seftor RE. Vasculogenic mimicry and tumour-cell plasticity: lessons from melanoma. Nat Rev Cancer. 2003;3(6):411–21.
16. Mittal K, Ebos J, Rini B. Angiogenesis and the tumor microenvironment: vascular endothelial growth factor and beyond. Semin Oncol. 2014;41(2):235–51.
17. Sennino B, McDonald DM. Controlling escape from angiogenesis inhibitors. Nat Rev Cancer. 2012;12(10):699–709.
18. Murdoch C, Muthana M, Coffelt SB, Lewis CE. The role of myeloid cells in the promotion of tumour angiogenesis. Nat Rev Cancer. 2008;8(8):618–31.
19. Pickup MW, Mouw JK, Weaver VM. The extracellular matrix modulates the hallmarks of cancer. EMBO Rep. 2014;15(12):1243–53.
20. Corrie PG, Basu B, Zaki KA. Targeting angiogenesis in melanoma: prospects for the future. Ther Adv Med Oncol. 2010;2(6):367–80.
21. Neufeld G, Cohen T, Gengrinovitch S, Poltorak Z. Vascular endothelial growth factor (VEGF) and its receptors. FASEB J Off Publ Federation Am Soc Exp Biol. 1999;13(1):9–22.
22. Chung HJ, Mahalingam M. Angiogenesis, vasculogenic mimicry and vascular invasion in cutaneous malignant melanoma – implications for therapeutic strategies and targeted therapies. Expert Rev Anticancer Ther. 2014;14(5):621–39.
23. Goel HL, Mercurio AM. VEGF targets the tumour cell. Nat Rev Cancer. 2013;13(12):871–82.
24. Gitay-Goren H, Halaban R, Neufeld G. Human melanoma cells but not normal melanocytes express vascular endothelial growth factor receptors. Biochem Biophys Res Commun. 1993;190(3):702–8.
25. Erhard H, Rietveld FJ, van Altena MC, Brocker EB, Ruiter DJ, de Waal RM. Transition of horizontal to vertical growth phase melanoma is accompanied by induction of vascular endothelial growth factor expression and angiogenesis. Melanoma Res. 1997;7(Suppl 2):S19–26.
26. Salven P, Heikkila P, Joensuu H. Enhanced expression of vascular endothelial growth factor in metastatic melanoma. Br J Cancer. 1997;76(7):930–4.
27. Chua R, Setzer S, Govindarajan B, Sexton D, Cohen C, Arbiser JL. Maspin expression, angiogenesis, prognostic parameters, and outcome in malignant melanoma. J Am Acad Dermatol. 2009;60(5):758–66.
28. Tas F, Duranyildiz D, Oguz H, Camlica H, Yasasever V, Topuz E. Circulating levels of vascular endothelial growth factor (VEGF), matrix metalloproteinase-3 (MMP-3), and BCL-2 in malignant melanoma. Med Oncol. 2008;25(4):431–6.
29. Hellberg C, Ostman A, Heldin CH. PDGF and vessel maturation. Recent results in cancer research Fortschritte der Krebsforschung. Progres dans les recherches sur le cancer. 2010;180:103–14.
30. Gaengel K, Genove G, Armulik A, Betsholtz C. Endothelial-mural cell signaling in vascular development and angiogenesis. Arterioscler Thromb Vasc Biol. 2009;29(5):630–8.
31. Barnhill RL, Xiao M, Graves D, Antoniades HN. Expression of platelet-derived growth factor (PDGF)-A, PDGF-B and the PDGF-alpha receptor, but not the PDGF-beta receptor, in human malignant melanoma in vivo. Br J Dermatol. 1996;135(6):898–904.

32. Halaban R, Ghosh S, Baird A. bFGF is the putative natural growth factor for human melano-cytes. In Vitro Cell Dev Biol J Tissue Culture Assoc. 1987;23(1):47–52.
33. Metzner T, Bedeir A, Held G, Peter-Vorosmarty B, Ghassemi S, Heinzle C, et al. Fibroblast growth factor receptors as therapeutic targets in human melanoma: synergism with BRAF inhibition. J Investigative Dermatology. 2011;131(10):2087–95.
34. Helfrich I, Edler L, Sucker A, Thomas M, Christian S, Schadendorf D, et al. Angiopoietin-2 levels are associated with disease progression in metastatic malignant melanoma. Clin Cancer Res Off J Am Assoc Cancer Res. 2009;15(4):1384–92.
35. Phng LK, Gerhardt H. Angiogenesis: a team effort coordinated by notch. Dev Cell. 2009;16(2):196–208.
36. Phng LK, Potente M, Leslie JD, Babbage J, Nyqvist D, Lobov I, et al. Nrarp coordinates endo-thelial Notch and Wnt signaling to control vessel density in angiogenesis. Dev Cell. 2009;16(1):70–82.
37. Folkman J. Tumor angiogenesis: therapeutic implications. N Engl J Med. 1971;285(21):1182–6.
38. Vasudev NS, Reynolds AR. Anti-angiogenic therapy for cancer: current progress, unresolved questions and future directions. Angiogenesis. 2014;17(3):471–94.
39. Bergers G, Hanahan D. Modes of resistance to anti-angiogenic therapy. Nat Rev Cancer. 2008;8(8):592–603.
40. Ferrara N, Hillan KJ, Gerber HP, Novotny W. Discovery and development of bevacizumab, an anti-VEGF antibody for treating cancer. Nat Rev Drug Discov. 2004;3(5):391–400.
41. Spaide RF, Laud K, Fine HF, Klancnik Jr JM, Meyerle CB, Yannuzzi LA, et al. Intravitreal bevacizumab treatment of choroidal neovascularization secondary to age-related macular degeneration. Retina. 2006;26(4):383–90.
42. Kim KB, Sosman JA, Fruehauf JP, Linette GP, Markovic SN, McDermott DF, et al. BEAM: a randomized phase II study evaluating the activity of bevacizumab in combination with carbo-platin plus paclitaxel in patients with previously untreated advanced melanoma. J Clin Oncol Off J Am Soc Clin Oncol. 2012;30(1):34–41.
43. Amit L, Ben-Aharon I, Vidal L, Leibovici L, Stemmer S. The impact of Bevacizumab (Avastin) on survival in metastatic solid tumors – a meta-analysis and systematic review. PLoS One. 2013;8(1):e51780.
44. Huang Y, Goel S, Duda DG, Fukumura D, Jain RK. Vascular normalization as an emerging strategy to enhance cancer immunotherapy. Cancer Res. 2013;73(10):2943–8.
45. Vihinen PP, Hernberg M, Vuoristo MS, Tyynela K, Laukka M, Lundin J, et al. A phase II trial of bevacizumab with dacarbazine and daily low-dose interferon-alpha2a as first line treatment in metastatic melanoma. Melanoma Res. 2010;20(4):318–25.
46. Grignol VP, Olencki T, Relekar K, Taylor C, Kibler A, Kefauver C, et al. A phase 2 trial of bevacizumab and high-dose interferon alpha 2B in metastatic melanoma. J Immunother. 2011;34(6):509–15.
47. Del Vecchio M, Mortarini R, Canova S, Di Guardo L, Pimpinelli N, Sertoli MR, et al. Bevacizumab plus fotemustine as first-line treatment in metastatic melanoma patients: clinical activity and modulation of angiogenesis and lymphangiogenesis factors. Clin Cancer Res Off J Am Assoc Cancer Res. 2010;16(23):5862–72.
48. Slingluff Jr CL, Petroni GR, Molhoek KR, Brautigan DL, Chianese-Bullock KA, Shada AL, et al. Clinical activity and safety of combination therapy with temsirolimus and bevacizumab for advanced melanoma: a phase II trial (CTEP 7190/Mel47). Clin Cancer Res Off J Am Assoc Cancer Res. 2013;19(13):3611–20.
49. von Moos R, Seifert B, Simcock M, Goldinger SM, Gillessen S, Ochsenbein A, et al. First-line temozolomide combined with bevacizumab in metastatic melanoma: a multicentre phase II trial (SAKK 50/07). Ann Oncol Off J Eur Soc Medical Oncol ESMO. 2012;23(2):531–6.
50. Kottschade LA, Suman VJ, Perez DG, McWilliams RR, Kaur JS, Amatruda 3rd TT, et al. A randomized phase 2 study of temozolomide and bevacizumab or nab-paclitaxel, carboplatin,

and bevacizumab in patients with unresectable stage IV melanoma: a North Central Cancer Treatment Group study, N0775. Cancer. 2013;119(3):586–92.

51. Ohm JE, Carbone DP. VEGF as a mediator of tumor-associated immunodeficiency. Immunol Res. 2001;23(2–3):263–72.

52. Oyama T, Ran S, Ishida T, Nadaf S, Kerr L, Carbone DP, et al. Vascular endothelial growth factor affects dendritic cell maturation through the inhibition of nuclear factor-kappa B activation in hemopoietic progenitor cells. J Immunol. 1998;160(3):1224–32.

53. Terme M, Pernot S, Marcheteau E, Sandoval F, Benhamouda N, Colussi O, et al. VEGFA-VEGFR pathway blockade inhibits tumor-induced regulatory T-cell proliferation in colorectal cancer. Cancer Res. 2013;73(2):539–49.

54. Gabrilovich DI, Ostrand-Rosenberg S, Bronte V. Coordinated regulation of myeloid cells by tumours. Nat Rev Immunol. 2012;12(4):253–68.

55. Terme M, Colussi O, Marcheteau E, Tanchot C, Tartour E, Taieb J. Modulation of immunity by antiangiogenic molecules in cancer. Clin Dev Immunol. 2012;2012:492920.

56. Hodi FS, Lawrence D, Lezcano C, Wu X, Zhou J, Sasada T, et al. Bevacizumab plus ipilimumab in patients with metastatic melanoma. Cancer Immunol Res. 2014;2(7):632–42.

57. Cameron D, Brown J, Dent R, Jackisch C, Mackey J, Pivot X, et al. Adjuvant bevacizumab-containing therapy in triple-negative breast cancer (BEATRICE): primary results of a randomised, phase 3 trial. Lancet Oncol. 2013;14(10):933–42.

58. Corrie PG, Marshall A, Dunn JA, Middleton MR, Nathan PD, Gore M, et al. Adjuvant bevacizumab in patients with melanoma at high risk of recurrence (AVAST-M): preplanned interim results from a multicentre, open-label, randomised controlled phase 3 study. Lancet Oncol. 2014;15(6):620–30.

59. Wu J, Brunner G, Celebi JT. A melanoma subtype: uveal melanoma. J Am Acad Dermatol. 2011;64(6):1185–6.

60. LoConte NK, Thomas JP, Alberti D, Heideman J, Binger K, Marnocha R, et al. A phase I pharmacodynamic trial of bortezomib in combination with doxorubicin in patients with advanced cancer. Cancer Chemother Pharmacol. 2008;63(1):109–15.

61. el Filali M, Ly LV, Luyten GP, Versluis M, Grossniklaus HE, van der Velden PA, et al. Bevacizumab and intraocular tumors: an intriguing paradox. Mol Vis. 2012;18:2454–67.

62. el Filali M, van der Velden PA, Luyten GP, Jager MJ. Anti-angiogenic therapy in uveal melanoma. Dev Ophthalmol. 2012;49:117–36.

63. Tarhini AA, Frankel P, Margolin KA, Christensen S, Ruel C, Shipe-Spotloe J, et al. Aflibercept (VEGF Trap) in inoperable stage III or stage iv melanoma of cutaneous or uveal origin. Clin Cancer Res Off J Am Assoc Cancer Res. 2011;17(20):6574–81.

64. Motzer RJ, Hutson TE, Tomczak P, Michaelson MD, Bukowski RM, Rixe O, et al. Sunitinib versus interferon alfa in metastatic renal-cell carcinoma. N Engl J Med. 2007;356(2):115–24.

65. Ahmad T, Eisen T. Kinase inhibition with BAY 43-9006 in renal cell carcinoma. Clin Cancer Res Off J Am Assoc Cancer Res. 2004;10(18 Pt 2):6388S–92S.

66. Demetri GD, van Oosterom AT, Garrett CR, Blackstein ME, Shah MH, Verweij J, et al. Efficacy and safety of sunitinib in patients with advanced gastrointestinal stromal tumour after failure of imatinib: a randomised controlled trial. Lancet. 2006;368(9544):1329–38.

67. Faivre S, Delbaldo C, Vera K, Robert C, Lozahic S, Lassau N, et al. Safety, pharmacokinetic, and antitumor activity of SU11248, a novel oral multitarget tyrosine kinase inhibitor, in patients with cancer. J Clin Oncol Off J Am Soc Clin Oncol. 2006;24(1):25–35.

68. Ishak RS, Aad SA, Kyei A, Farhat FS. Cutaneous manifestations of anti-angiogenic therapy in oncology: review with focus on VEGF inhibitors. Crit Rev Oncol Hematol. 2014;90(2):152–64.

Potential Role of Angiogenesis and Lymphangiogenesis in Atopic Dermatitis: Evidence from Human Studies and Lessons from an Animal Model of Human Disease

6

Huayi Zhang, Vivian Y. Shi, and Lawrence S. Chan

Abbreviations

AD	Atopic dermatitis
ANG-1	Angiopoeitin-1
ANG-2	Angiopoeitin-2
BO	Before onset
CAM	Cell adhesion molecule
EB	Evans Blue
EC	Endothelial cell
EL	Early lesion
FGF-β	Fibroblast growth factor-beta
HaCaT	Human adult high calcium low temperature keratinoctyes
IEJC	Interendothelial junctional cleft
IgSF CAMs	Immunoglobulin super family cell adhesion molecules
K14	Keratin-14
LECs	Lymphatic endothelial cells
LL	Late lesion
LYVE-1	Lymphatic vessel endothelial hyaluronan receptor

H. Zhang, MD • V.Y. Shi, MD
Department of Dermatology, University of Illinois College of Medicine,
MC624, R380, 808 S Wood, Chicago 60612, IL, USA

L.S. Chan, MD (✉)
Department of Dermatology, University of Illinois College of Medicine,
MC624, R380, 808 S Wood, Chicago 60612, IL, USA

Department of Microbiology/Immunology, University of Illinois College of Medicine,
Chicago, IL, USA

Medicine Services, Jesse Brown VA Medical Center, Chicago, IL, USA

Captain James Lovell Federal Health Care Center, North Chicago, IL, USA
e-mail: larrycha@uic.edu

© Springer-Verlag London Ltd. 2017
J.L. Arbiser (ed.), *Angiogenesis-Based Dermatology*,
DOI 10.1007/978-1-4471-7314-4_6

MCP-1	Macrophage chemotactic protein-1
NRP-1,2	Neuropilin-1,2
NT	Non-transgenic
PAR$_2$	Proteinase-activated receptor 2
PECAM-1	Platelet endothelial cell adhesion molecule-1
PCV	Dermal post-capillary venules
PDPN	Podoplanin
SEM	Scanning electronic microscopy
SNPs	Single nucleotide polymorphisms
TEM	Transitional electron microscopy
Tg	Transgenic
TJ	Tight junction
VAP-1	Vascular adhesion protein-1
VEGF-A, B, C, D	Vascular endothelial cell growth factor-A, B, C, D
VEGFR-1, 2, 3	Vascular endothelial cell growth factor receptor-1, 2, 3

Introduction

Atopic dermatitis (AD) is a chronic recurring skin condition manifested clinically by inflammation, intense pruritus and marked by cycles of exacerbations and remissions. As defined by the United Kingdom's refined diagnostic criteria for epidemiologic studies (Table 6.1), a diagnosis of AD should fulfill at least 1 major criteria of having a pruritic skin condition lasting at least 12 months and 3 minor criteria [1]. The disease can affect both genders equally at all ages but occurs more frequently during infancy. In the United States, it is estimated that 65% of patients develop symptoms in their first year of life, and 80% develop symptoms before the age of 5 [2]. Although the symptoms of AD resolve by adolescence in 50% of affected children, the condition persists into adulthood in about half of these patients. Data also suggests that AD patients have a higher incidence of developing asthma, hay fever and food allergies [3]. The progression of these allergic diseases often begin with AD in early childhood. About one half to two thirds of AD patients subsequently "march on" to develop asthma and allergic rhinitis, respectively, as suggested by the term "atopic march" [4]. The "atopic march" theory is based on the idea that the skin overwhelmed with allergens will increase the migration of T-cells into the airways, leading to upper and lower respiratory tract infections [4]. AD has also become a common cause of workplace disability with increasing medical expenditure. AD Worldwide, the prevalence of AD has increased over the past decade with the problem more acutely seen in developing nations. In a recent analysis of medical expenditure in the United States, it is estimated that both direct costs (doctor visits, hospitalizations, and medicine) and indirect costs (over-the-counter remedies, and days lost from work) for AD may exceed $3 billion annually, placing a huge burden on the US healthcare system [2].

Table 6.1 The United Kingdom's refined diagnostic criteria for atopic dermatitis

Major criteria (Required for diagnosis)
Any pruritic skin condition in the past 12 months
Minor criteria (Require 3 of the following)
Age of onset younger than 2 years[a]
History of flexural skin involvement
History of generalized dry skin
Personal history of other atopic disease[b]
Clinical flexural dermatitis documented by photographic protocol

Reproduced with permission, Chan et al. [1]
[a]Not used for children younger than 4 years
[b]For children younger than 4 years, history of atopic disease in a first degree relative may be used

Although the pathogenesis of AD remains to be fully deciphered, this multifactorial disease is likely a product of both genetic and environmental factors. Data from human and animal studies indicate that a Th2 cell immune response is dominant during the acute phase of AD, and that a Th1 cell response is prevalent during the chronic phase [5–7]. In addition, infiltration of inflammatory cells, defective epidermis barrier functions, and high levels of inflammatory mediators are typically associated with AD [5, 6]. The current approach towards the management of AD has mainly been to suppress the inflammatory nature of the disease. Although this approach helps to control the inflammation and the symptoms of AD, it does not cure the chronic problem.

Recent studies of factors involved in inflammatory disease have focused on angiogenesis and lymphangiogenesis. The process of neovascularization has been found to be important in other inflammatory disorders like rheumatoid arthritis, psoriasis and some autoimmune diseases [8]. Since blood vessels are the essential pathways for transporting immune cells (T cells, eosinophils, dendritic cells and macrophages) to the site of inflammation, examining the role of vasculature in the inflammatory skin diseases seems to be a logical approach. Pro-inflammatory mediators such as selectins, cell adhesion molecules (CAM), integrins, cytokines, chemokines, as well as vascular endothelial growth factors (VEGF), have been associated with the process of new capillary formation. As angiogenesis and lymphangiogenesis are the development of microvasculature in response to inflammatory agents, these two phenomena could in theory play some roles in the pathogenesis of AD - as AD is a prototypic chronic inflammatory disease [9].

Currently, there is a scarcity of research studies that demonstrate angiogenesis or lymphangiogenesis in human AD. In the following sections, our review on human AD will be primarily on the role of vasculature in AD development. We will then review the strong evidence of angiogenesis and lymphangiogenesis in an animal model of AD. By understanding the potential roles of vasculature and neovascularization in AD, we may be able to open a novel path to therapeutic intervention.

Evidence of Angiogenesis and Lymphangiogenesis in Human Atopic Dermatitis

Selectins

The early steps of the inflammatory process involves leukocyte extravasation. Evidence suggests that upon antigenic stimulation, resident macrophages in the affected tissue release cytokines and chemokines such as IL-1 and TNFα and CCL-5 which attract circulating leukocytes to the site of injury. TNF alpha and IFN gamma then induce the endothelial cells at the activated site to express adhesion molecules called selectins. These molecules allow for the tethering and adhesion of leukocytes to the vascular endothelium [10]. Upon stimulation, L-selectin, found on all circulating leukocytes, and E- and P-selectins, expressed on the activated endothelial cells, will bind to each other's complementary carbohydrate ligands with marginal affinity. This will facilitate the process of rolling and tethering of the leukocytes along the inner surface of the blood vessel walls. Research has indeed shown that E-selectin levels are elevated in lesional skin of adults and children with AD [11]. There is also a positive correlation between the number of mononuclear cells and T cells with the degree of E-selectin expression in lesioned skin of human AD [11]. In the CD4 T cells of AD patients, an increase in L-selectin level was also detected [12]. Because of this data, selectin levels have been suggested as a biomarker for AD disease activity as well as treatment response [13].

Immunoglobulin Superfamily Cell Adhesion Molecules

Another subset of the cellular adhesion molecules are a large group of cell surface proteins involved in the recognition and binding of cells known as the immuno-globulin superfamily cell adhesion molecules (IgSF CAMs). These proteins have domains that are similar in structure to antibodies and can activate leukocytes, thereby enhancing their adhesion to other leukocytes and endothelial cells. The IgSF on endothelial cells, ICAM-1, 2, 3 and VCAM-1 are expressed at different phases of the inflammatory process and bind to their respective β2 integrin ligands to initiate adhesion [12]. While VCAM-1 and ICAM-1 are minimally expressed in the blood vessels of non-atopic individuals, they are strongly expressed in the non-lesional skin and expressed with greater intensity in lesional skin of AD patients, suggesting their involvement in the inflammatory process [14].

New cell adhesion molecules have emerged in the study of AD pathophysiology. One molecule of interest is the vascular adhesion protein-1 (VAP-1), which was discovered in the late 1980s to be involved in the inflammation of arthritis as well as in lymphocyte migration in inflamed skin and the gut [15]. It also participates in the adhesion cascade of multiple tissues by allowing the lymphocyte-endothelial cell interaction to occur. One study showed that VAP-1 was overexpressed in both the lesional and non-lesional skin biopsies of AD patients. The fact that the serum levels of VAP-1 decreased after AD therapy also suggests a role of VAP-1 in the AD disease process [15].

Integrins

Mechanistically, certain chemokines released by macrophages could cause cellular transmembrane receptor molecules integrins to switch from a low-affinity state to a high-affinity state. Once activated, integrins will bind tightly to complementary receptors expressed on vascular endothelial cells with high affinity allowing for a firm attachment of the leukocytes. This action functions to prevent WBCs from being swept away by the shear forces of the ongoing blood flow. Similarly, integrins on eosinophils' cell surface can also recognize the laminin, fibronectin, and glycos-aminoglycans hyaluronic acid of the extracellular matrix allowing the eosinophils to firmly attach to the sites of inflammation [16]. Of note, the $\alpha 6$ integrin, found on the luminal side of blood vessels, have been studied for its role in binding migratory T cells in atopic skin. A significant up-regulation of the $\alpha 6$ integrin has been found on the endothelial cells and in the epidermis of lesional skin of AD as compared to control, supporting a role of this integrin in the inflammatory process of AD [17].

Transmigration

The entire process of diapedesis, the transmigration of the leukocytes out of the blood vessels, is well coordinated between leukocytes and endothelial cells. After adhesion to the endothelial cells, leukocytes rearrange their cytoskeleton so that they can flatten and spread out over the endothelium. In this morphology, leukocytes can extend their pseudopods and pass through the gaps created between neighboring endothelial cells. Platelet endothelial cell adhesion molecules (PECAM-1) proteins found on both leukocytes and endothelial cells can facilitate the movement of the leukocytes out of the endothelium [17]. Transmigration of the leukocyte continues with breaking through the basement membrane by way of either proteolytic digestion of the membrane and or mechanical forces. Once in the interstitium, leukocytes resume their travels towards the site of injury or infection via chemotactic agents. Significantly, the expression of PECAM-1 is highly increased in the lesional skin of AD patients as compared to uninvolved atopic skin [18].

Growth Factors in Angiogenesis and AD

Growth factors involved in vascular remodeling have been identified with inflammatory disorders [19]. One growth factor of interest in inflammation-mediated angiogenesis is the vascular endothelial growth factor (VEGF), which is present in four different isoforms (A, B, C and D). As the name suggests, VEGF promotes the growth, survival and migration of endothelial cells and is a potent vasodilator. The A and B isoforms are angiogenic in nature with VEGF-A being the most pro-angiogentic isoform, while the C and D isoforms are involved in lymphangiogenesis [20]. VEGF signals through three human VEGF receptors (VEGFR-1,2,3) [21] and two co-receptors, Neuropilin-1, 2 (NRP-1,2) [22]. NRP-1 is mainly expressed on arterial endothelial cells and has the binding affinity for VEGF-A [23]. NPR-2 is found on venous and lymphatic endothelial cells [24], thereby supporting lymphan-giogenesis. By changing the vascular permeability, remodeling the vascular tone, and increasing blood flow and surface area to promote leukocyte-endothelial cell interactions, VEGF contributes to the angiogenic process. Its increased expression in the epidermis of AD patients has been documented [25]. The ability to increase blood vessel dilation and permeability, as well as being a chemotactic factor for monocytes, may make VEGF a key participant of inflammatory disease in general and of AD onset and development in particular [26]. In fact, researchers confirmed that the levels of the stratum corneum VEGF not only correlated with the disease severity but also with the levels of serum LDH and the amount of eosinophils in AD patients [25].

It has been suggested that single nucleotide polymorphisms (SNPs) may be asso-ciated with VEGF overexpression. Shahbazi et al. showed that at position 1154 on chromosome 6p12, the GG and GA genotypes of the VEGF gene is linked to higher VEGF production by mononuclear cells [27]. By digging deeper into gene poly-morphism, other have discovered that AD patients have greater GA expression at position 1154 of the promoter region of the VEGF gene which may be accounted for the higher levels of VEGF expression.

Mediators Involved in Angiogenesis and AD

Mast cells

Increasing experimental evidence suggests that inflammatory cells contribute to the development of AD by creating angiogenic and lymphangiogenic factors. Human mast cells are a likely contributor because of their close proximity to epidermal endothelial cells and because of their abilities to release pro-angiogenic factors and histamine which can trigger increased vascular permeability, smooth muscle con-tractions and vasodilation. Investigators have demonstrated that human skin mast cells, which are abundant in the lesional skin of AD patients, contain and release VEGF-A, B, C and D as well as the various VEGFR, thereby serving both as a source and a target for VEGF. [28] From this observation, it was postulated that the VEGF made by the mast cells can recruit more mast cells to the site of inflammation in a paracrine fashion in order to sustain the angiogenic process in AD. [20]

Mast cells are also known to release tryptase, an enzyme that can activate the receptor proteinase-activated receptor 2 (PAR$_2$) on the dermal endothelium result-ing in the up-regulation of ICAM-1 and E-selectin. The levels of tryptase and PAR$_2$ are observed to be elevated in the lesional skin of AD patients suggesting localized mast cell involvement in skin inflammation. [29]

The close proximity of epidermal and papillary mast cells to endothelial cells may allow mast cells to participate in cutaneous inflammation and angiogenesis. CD31-positive endothelial cells were found to grow only in the company of surrounding mast cells from the papillae up to the stratum granulosum. Even more interestingly, mast cells may exhibit a bidirectional "tunneling" effect in the epidermis of AD patients. In the "forward" direction, mast cells secrete matrix-degrading enzymes like MMPs which clears out a tunnel in the epidermis. While in the "backwards" direction, mast cells secrete pro-angiogenic factors, so that new vessels can be attracted to sprout into the tunnel behind it. [30] In fact experiments have shown an increase in MMP-2 expression along with several pro-angiogenic factors in the presence of mast cells in AD skin. [30]

Cytokines

Cytokines and endothelial cells are co-factors in inflammation. Various interleukins, such as IL-1, 4, 6, 8, 9 and 17, have been identified with special contributions to vascular regulation and AD. [12, 31] IL-1 and TNF-alpha both up-regulate ICAM-1 and E-selectin, resulting in the activation of dermal vascular endothelial cells. IL-17 further augments this effect by inducing more IL-1 secretion from the same endothelial cells. IL-17 also enhances the actions of fibroblast growth factor-beta (FGF-β) and VEGF, stimulating angiogenesis and endothelial cell migration. [32]

IL-4 plays an important role in the pathogenesis of AD. It has been shown to up-regulate AD related chemokines CCL25, CCL26, pro-inflammatory factors IL-1, IL-19 and IL-20 as well the pro-angiogenic factor VEGFA in human keratinocytes [31], thus providing a link between angiogenesis and atopic dermatitis.

Various studies have cited that AD patients have increased levels of IL-8 in the plasma and eosinophils. IL-8 is also known to mediate angiogenesis by increasing endothelial cell proliferation and chemotaxis. [20]

IL-9 was initially defined as a T-cell and mast cell growth factor associated with the Th2 immune response. It has only recently been reported to promote VEGF release from mast cells through STAT3 activation. [33] IL-9 and IL-9 receptor mRNA expressions are in fact highly elevated in the lesioned skin of AD patients as compared with controls. [33] These data are revealing of IL-9's role in both angiogenesis and AD.

IL-6 is a well-known mediator of inflammation and is produced by endothelial cells. IL-6 in turn acts on endothelial cells to further increase their growth and activation. Up-regulation of IL-6 is not only found in human AD but can cause inflammation in various other diseases. [12]

Chemokines

Chemokines are involved in both the adhesion and trans-membrane migration segments of the leukocyte extravasation process in the endothleium. In AD, endothelial cells, keratinocytes, and fibroblasts can provide a variety of chemokines to attract leukocytes. [12] For example, chemokines such as CCL11, CCL13, CCL17, CCL18, CCL22, CCL26 and CCL27 have higher expression in the skin of AD patients as compared to normal subjects. [34] CCL-1, 11 and 26 can interact with endothelial cells to stimulate angiogenesis leading to further exacerbation. [12]

Evidence of Angiogenesis and Hymphangiogenesis in a Mouse Model of Atopic Dermatitis

Generation and Characterization of the Model

Since studies of angiogenesis and lymphangiogenesis in human AD are limited in scope and in depth, we next examine the evidence from an animal model. Developed in 2001 by Chan et al., the Keratin-14-IL-4 Transgenic (IL-4 Tg) mouse line is the only known AD experimental animal model with characteristic chronic inflammation. [35] The IL-4 Tg mouse was established by over-expression of IL-4, a critical Th2 cytokine involved in AD pathogenesis, in epidermal keratinocytes using a Keratin-14 promoter/enhancer. The IL-4 Tg mice spontaneously developed pathologic phenotypes that fulfilled key diagnostic criteria of AD seen in human patients. [36] Clinically, the Tg mice developed xerosis and pruritic inflammatory lesions in the ears starting at age of 4 months. Lesions later extend to the neck, mouth, eyes, back, torso, tail and legs (Fig. 6.1). Eye involvement caused eyelid dermatitis, blepharitis and conjunctivitis frequently result in corneal and conjunctival scarring. Microbiologically, crusted lesions and bacterial pyoderma developed at the external ears from self-excoriation are culture-positive for *Staphylococccus aureus* and *Pseudomonas aeruginosa*, with the former being a common infectious agent leading to disease exacerbation in human AD patients. Histopathologically, when compared to Non-transgenic (NT) littermates, the Tg mice skin lesions are characterized by increased spongiosis, acanthosis, and prominent epidermal and dermal infiltration of CD3+ T cells, macrophage-like mononuclear cells, degranulating mast cells, and eosinophils (Fig. 6.2). Despite epidermal over-expression of IL-4, the serum IL-4 level remains undetectable by ELISA. Immunologically, the onset and severity of skin disease correlate with the elevation and maintenance of serum levels of total IgE and IgG1. To monitor the disease progression and to correlate its progression with immunological mechanism, the Tg mice are classified into three groups based on disease progression, Tg-BO for mice before onset of any visible skin lesion,

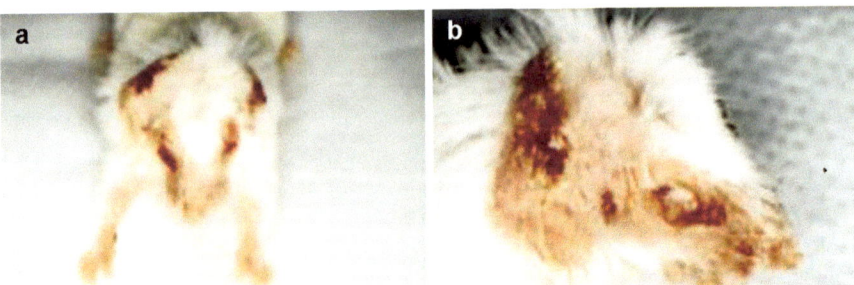

Fig. 6.1 Clinical manifestation of atopic dermatitis in affected IL-4 Tg mouse. Severe dermatitis on head and neck with areas of crusting, hair loss and bacterial pyoderma (**a**). External ear destruction results from self-excoriation and eyelid dermatitis leads to corneal and conjunctival scarring (**b**) (Reproduced with permission, Chan et al. [35])

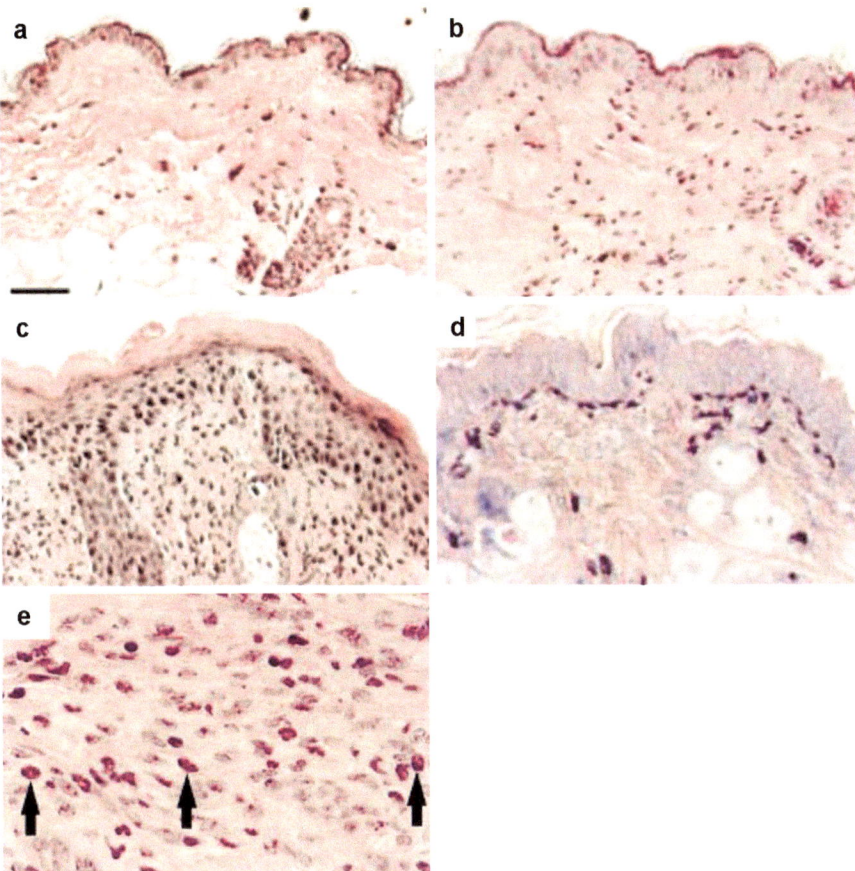

Fig. 6.2 Histopathological findings of skin lesions. NT littermates (**a**) have normal epidermal thickness with rare mononuclear cells. The skin of EL IL-4 Tg mice demonstrates mild spongiosis and acanthosis, with mononuclear cell infiltrate (**b**). LL mice demonstrate characteristics of chronic inflammatory lesion, with prominent hyperkeratosis and dermal mononuclear infiltrate, spongiosis and focal areas of parakeratosis (**c**). Mast cell degranulation (**d**) and eosinophil infiltrates (**e**) are also prominently present in chronic lesions. Hematoxylin & eosin (**a–c, e**). Geimsa (**d**) (Reproduced with permission, Chan et al. [35])

Tg-EL for mice with early/acute skin lesions of less than 1 week duration, and Tg-LL for mice with late/chronic skin lesions of equal to or greater than 3 weeks of duration.

Morphological Evidence

Angiogenesis occur in conjunction lymphangiogenesis in wound healing, inflammatory diseases such as peritonitis and rheumatoid arthritis. Dermal angiogenesis parallel lymphangiogenesis in psoriasis [37], a prototypic chronic inflammatory skin disease. However, limited data exist on the alteration of skin microcirculation of AD in human. Fueled by the successful introduction of the K14-IL-4 Tg mouse, much progress has been made to investigate the presence and pathogenic role of microvascular new growth in AD. First let us examine the morphological evidence.

Immunofluorescence Microscopic Evidence

Recent morphological studies revealed that both dermal angiogenesis and lymphangiogenesis are prominent features of the IL-4-Tg mouse. When compared to NT, the Tg mice have significantly higher expression of CD31 (an endothelial cell specific marker), and VEGFR-2 (VEGF receptor specific to blood vessels) per linear skin length. Furthermore, the average blood vessel diameter and skin area occupied by vessels increased as disease evolved from Tg-BO to Tg-EL and then to Tg-LL [38] (Fig. 6.3). Under confocal microscopy, Tg-EL and Tg-LL have increased dermal CD31 expression and reduced expression of claudin-5, an endothelial tight junction protein, when compared to NT and Tg-BO. This finding supports the notion that lesional skin has larger number of newly formed vessels, which characteristically have fewer tight junctions [39].

Identification of lymphatic vessel-specific markers in recent years enabled the study of inflammatory lymphangiogenesis. Dermal lymphangiogenesis parallels angiogenesis in the Tg mice. Lymphatic vessel-specific markers, such as podoplanin (PDPN), lymphatic vessel hyaluronan receptor (LYVE-1) and vascular endothelial cell growth factor receptor-3 (VEGFR-3) expressions were significantly increased in Tg mice when compared to NT mice [40] (Fig. 6.4). This phenomenon is observed even in lesion-free areas of the skin of the Tg mice. As seen in angiogenesis, the extent of lymphatic marker over-expression also correlates closely with disease severity, i.e., the severer the disease stage, the greater expression of lymphytic marker. When compared to NT littermates, the lymphatic vessels in Tg mice were greater in number, larger average and maximum diameter, and occupied more volume in the dermis. The evidence that the growth of both blood and lymphatic vessels match closely with the progression of skin lesions in Tg mice suggests a tight link between inflammatory reaction and neovascularization.

Electron Microscopic Evidence

Electron microscopy (EM) studies on the skin of the Tg mice revealed important ultrastructural changes in the microvascular beds [39]. Under transitional electron microscopy (TEM), the perivascular dermal matrix of NT mice consists of fibroblasts, collage and mast cells. NT mice have dermal blood capillaries that are continuous and formed by 1-2 endothelial cells (EC) with regular and smooth surfaces (Fig. 6.5a). In contrast, Tg mice dermal EC exhibit progressive nucleoli hypertrophy, cytoplasmic vacuolation, organelle hyperplasia, and increase in cell surface irregularity, thus demonstrating an endothelial cell activation process (Fig. 6.5b–d).

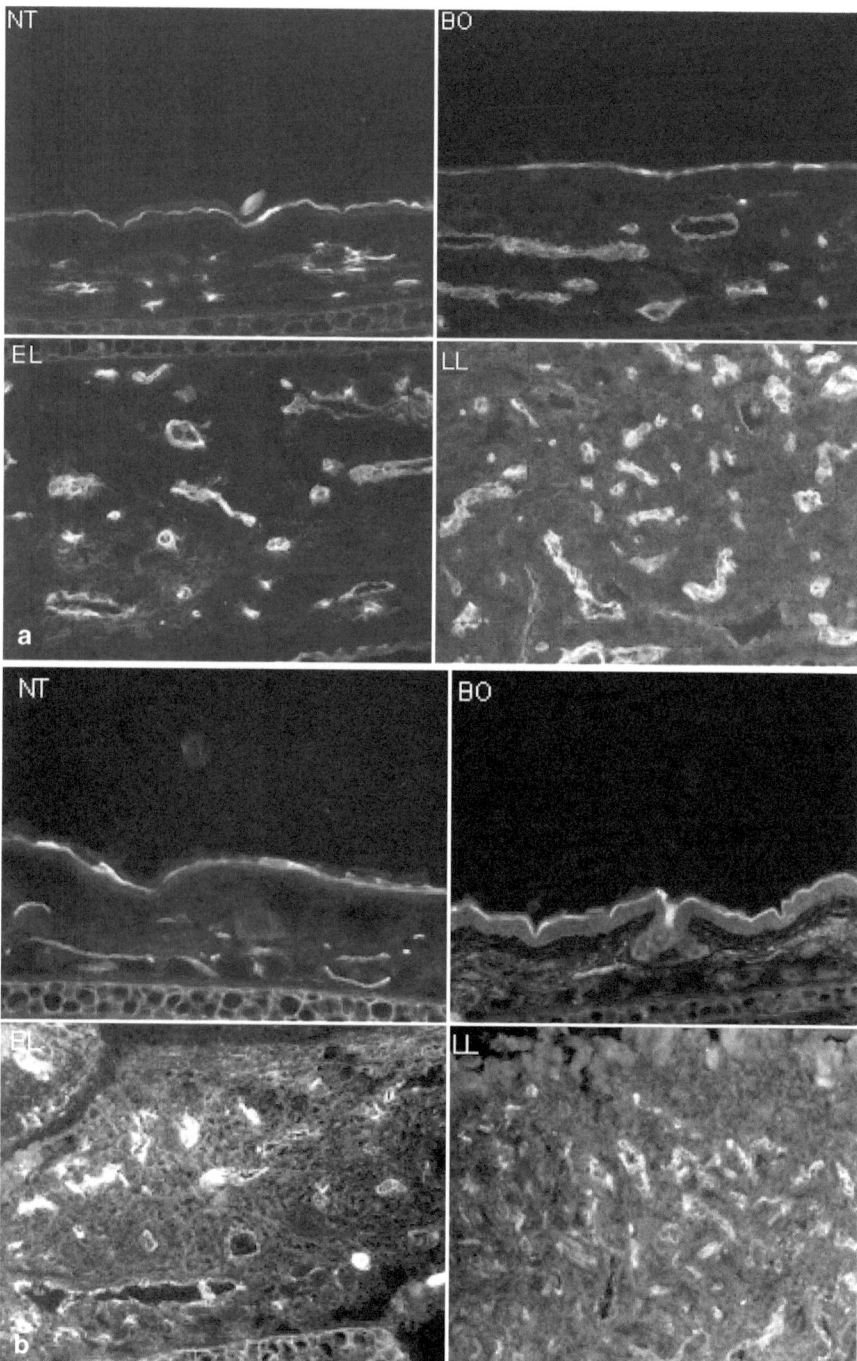

Fig. 6.3 Immunoflouresence microscopy of dermal vasculatures. CD31 (endothelial cell marker, Panel **a**) and VEGFR2 (VEGF receptor 2, Panel **b**) expressions parallel the severity of skin inflammation in the IL-4 Tg mouse. *Top left*, NT; *top right*, BO; *bottom left*, EL; *bottom right*, LL (Reproduced with permission, Chen et al. [38])

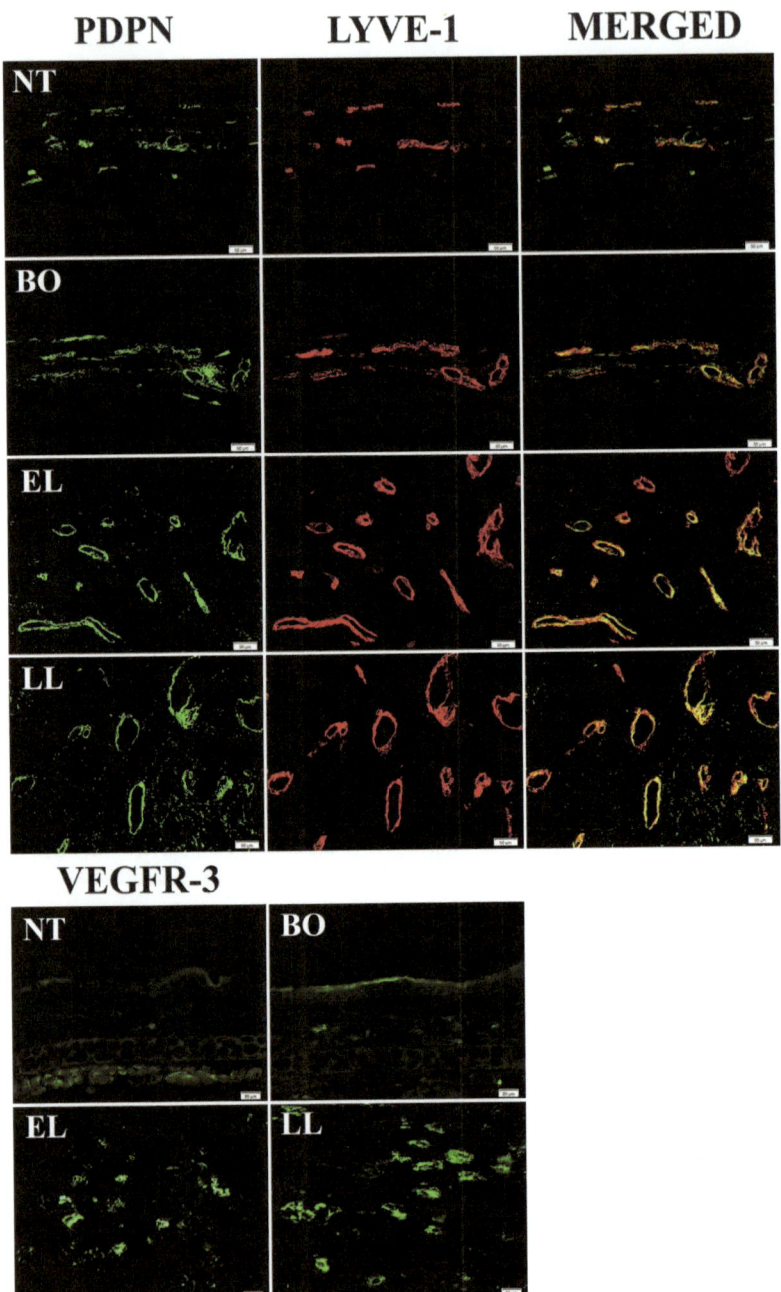

Fig. 6.4 Immunoflourescence microscopy of dermal lymphatics. Lymphatic- specific markers, *PDPN, LYVE-1* and *VEGFR-3* expressions are significantly increased in Tg mice when compared to NT mice. The increased expression of these three markers correlates with disease severity. *Left block*: PDPN (*green*) and LYVE-1 (*red*) co-localize on lymphatic endothelium (*merged*). *Right block*: VEGFR-3 expression in various disease stages. PDPN, podoplanin; LYVE-1 (lymphatic vessel hyaluronan receptor); VEGFR-3, vascular endothelial growth factor-3 (Reproduced with permission, Shi et al. [40])

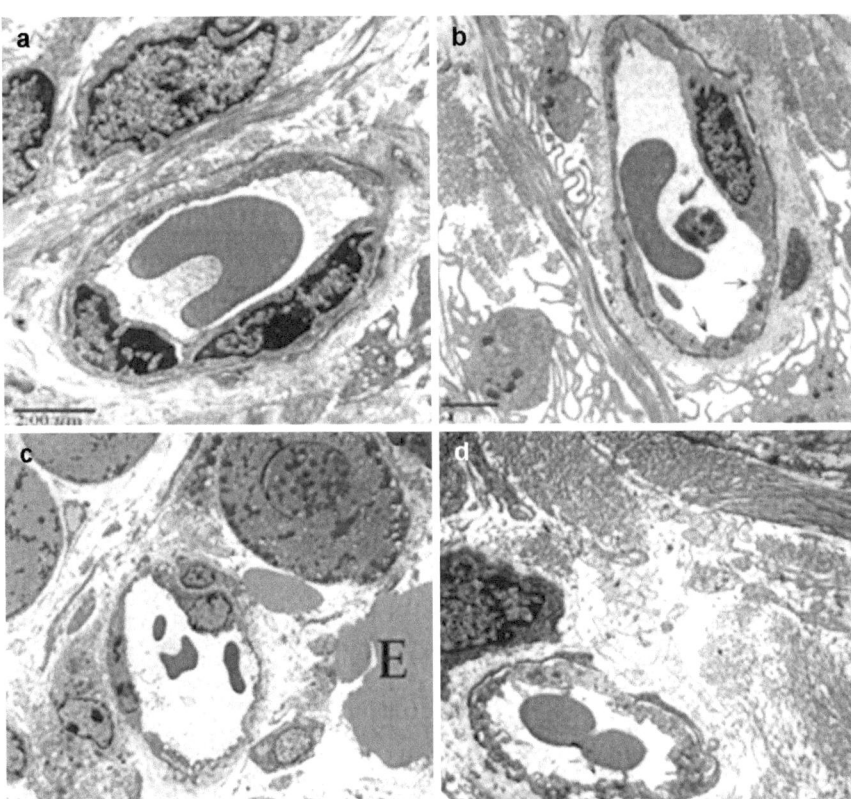

Fig.6.5 TEM micrographs of dermal capillaries. Capillaries of the NT mouse has thin continuous endothelium with regular and smooth surfaces (**a**). The capillaries of the IL-4 Tg mouse at BO stage still has continuous endothelium, but are thicker, more irregular and vacuolated. The endothelial cell (EC) nucleus is enlarged with prominent nucleoli, a sign of EC activation in preparation for angiogenesis (**b**). As disease progresses from EL (**c**) to LL (**d**) the capillary endothelium becomes increasingly irregular and vacuolated; ECs become increasingly hypertrophic with large nuclei and nucleoli and enlarged cytoplasm (Reproduced with permission, Agha-Majzoub et al. [39])

The extracellular matrix is also more edematous with increased erythrocyte extravasation. These ultrastructural alterations documented in the Tg mice are hallmarks of angiogenesis.

Endothelial remodeling is the fundamental process responsible to angiogenesis and we also examined this process by EM in AD. Angiogenic capillaries are distinguished from nonangiogenic capillaries by the presence of hypertrophied endothelial cells that appears activated with organelle rich cytoplasm and a minuscule lumen. In lesional skin of Tg mice, newly formed blood vessels form by intussusception, where interposition of transcapillary pillars allows division of one capillary into two separate capillaries (Fig. 6.6), whereas such observation is absent in NT mice. In Tg-EL and Tg-LL mice, both angiogenic and non-angiogenic capillaries were present.

Fig. 6.6 TEM showing capillary formation by intussusception during angiogenesis. New vessels form by the interposition of transcapillary pillars (*arrows*), which divides one capillary into two or more separate capillaries (Reproduced with permission, Agha-Majzoub et al. [39])

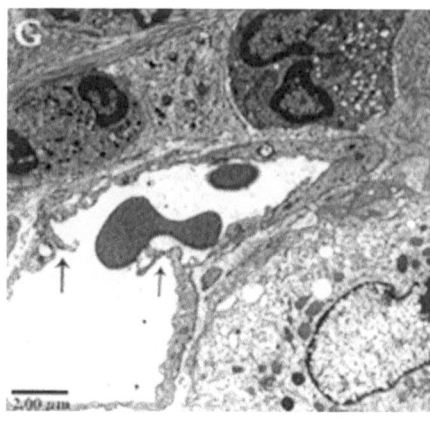

The angiogenic capillaries in EL have increased interendothelial junctional cleft (IEJC) length when compared to NT and BO (Fig. 6.7a–c), suggesting that angiogenic capillaries may adhere to each other by overlapping their plasma membrane surface. The elongated IEJC serves to provide surface area for new EC formation during angiogenesis.

The length ratio of tight junction (TJ) to IEJC was decreased in dermal postcapillary venules (PCV) and angiogenic capillaries in the EL and LL disease stages, when compared to that of BO stage and NT mice. This decrease in TJ: IEJC may be explained by a combination of IEJC length increase and reduction in TJ protein with disease progression. As the endothelial cells prepare to separate from each other in preparation for angiogenesis, IEJC increase in number and may transforms from simple, paracellular clefts seen in the skin of NT mice and Tg mice in BO stage (Fig. 6.7a, b) into the more complex, convoluted and interdigitated clefts in the skin of mice in EL and LL stages (Fig. 6.7c, d). TJ protein reduction is supported by the decrease in the expression of claudin-5, a TJ protein. Decreased TJ correlates with increased microvascular permeability and the emergence of fenestrations in EL and LL disease stages, a hallmark of skin inflammation and response to increased VEGF.

Furthermore, scanning electronic microscopy (SEM) provides a unique three-dimensional examination of vessels. The vascular bed of EL and LL mice appears strikingly different from NT mice. In NT mice and Tg mice in BO stage, the dermal microvasculature appears to have regular frame works consisted of smoothly organized branching pattern with scantly distributed vessels (Fig. 6.8a, b). The vessels branches in NT and BO mice often form near right angles. The vascular bed of BO mice shows early signs of vessel bedding, evidenced by subtle protrusions off the vessels, which may correspond to the disruption of JC seen in TEM (Fig. 6.8b). The vascular bed of EL and LL stages appear strikingly different from that of NT and BO mice. Both arteries and venules of the diseased mice in EL and LL stages become progressively torturous with increasing disease severity. EL and LL mice have more abundant and disorganized capillaries forming dense, sprouting endocasts. The capillaries of LL mice have the greatest heterogeneity, with highly

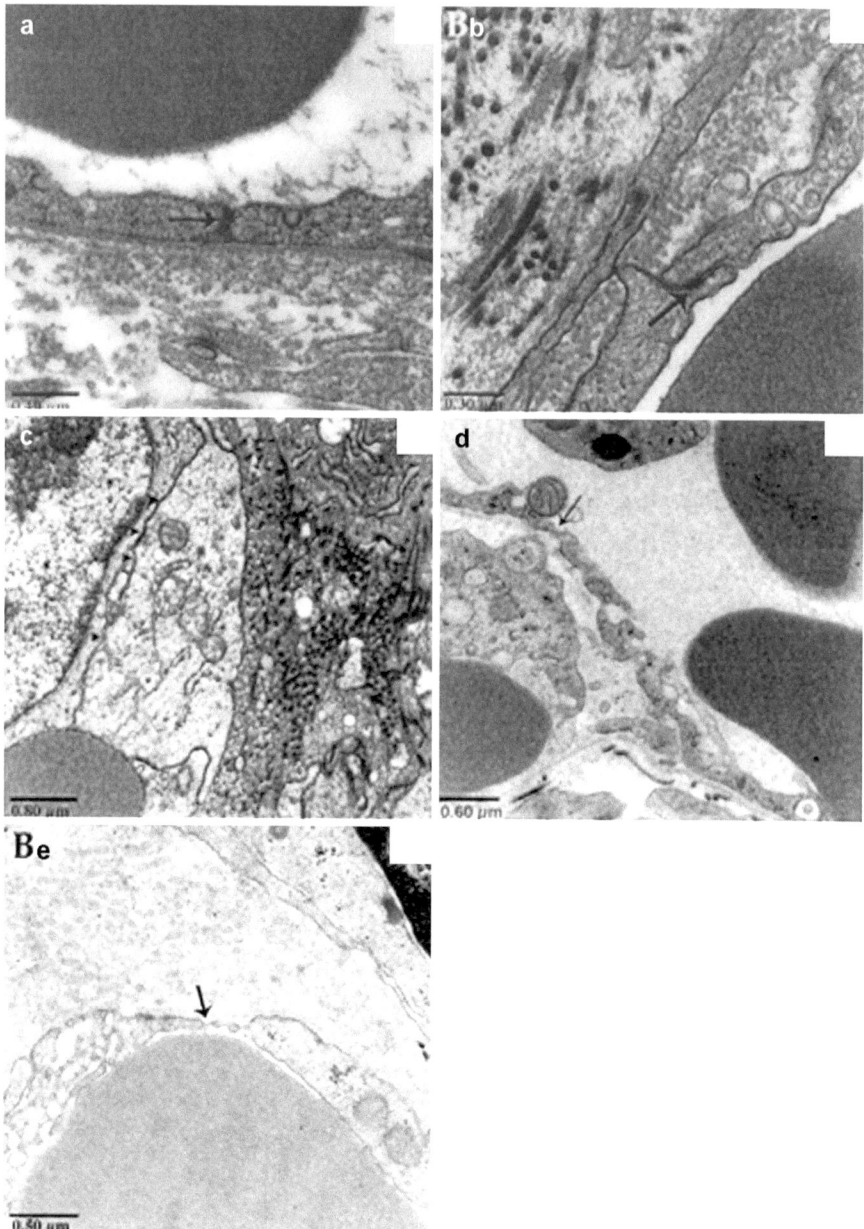

Fig. 6.7 TEM showing IEJC NT and IL-4 Tg mice. *Top row*: The dermal capillaries of the NT (**a**) and BO (**b**) mice have simple, short, and nonconvoluted IEJC; TJ located on the luminal aspect (*arrow*) (**a, b**). The IEJCs in EL are elongated (arrowheads) compared to those of BO and NT mice; TJs are located more towards to abluminal aspect of the IEJC compared to NT mouse (**c**). *Bottom row*: Endothelial cell fenestration are seen in the EL (**d**) and LL groups (**e**). IEJC, inter-endothelial junctional cleft; TJ, tight junction (Reproduced with permission, Agha-Majzoub et al. [39])

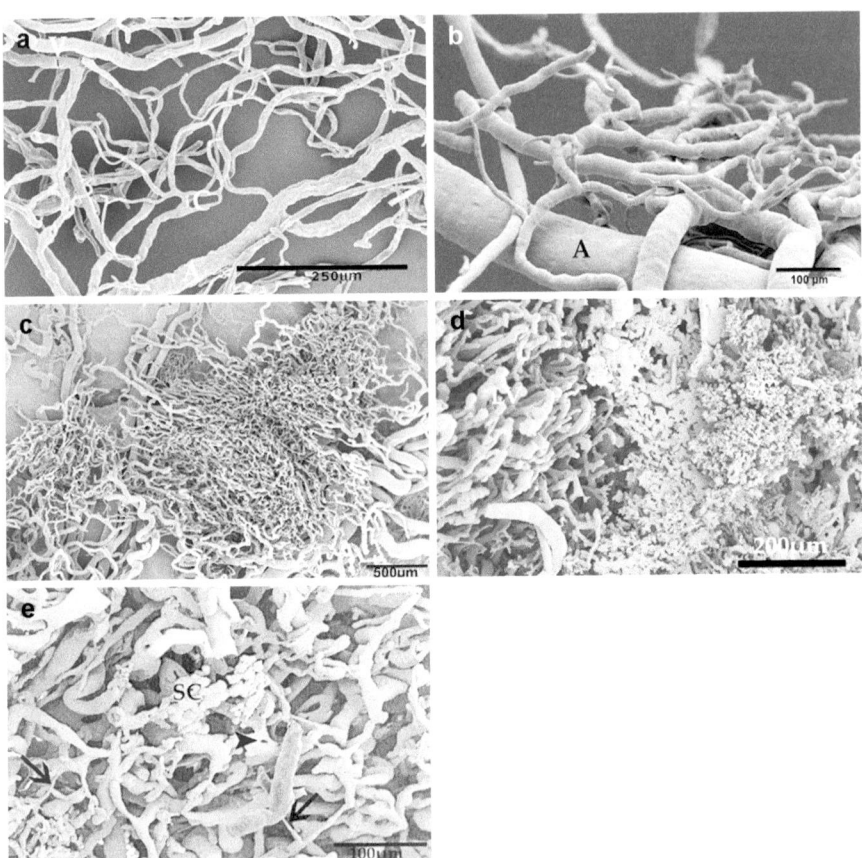

Fig. 6.8 SEM of the cast microvasculature in IL-4 Tg mice. The capillary network of NT (**a**) and BO (**b**) mice are low density and well organized. The vascular network of EL mouse appears more abundant, torturous and disorganized (**c**). In LL, the endocasts become very dense with no visible background (**d**). In higher magnification, the heterogenous blood vessels in the LL group has variable diameter (**e**). Small capillaries with bulbous sprouting (SC) and small extensions (*arrow*) are characteristics of angiogenesis (**e**) (Adapted with permission, Agha-Majzoub et al. [39])

irregular vascular diameter and surfaces. In contrast to those seen in NT and BO mice, the capillaries of LL mice form sharp angles as the disorganized vessels twist among each other (Fig. 6.8c, d). The center of the vasculature in LL consist of small capillaries forming bulbous sprouting, while sharply angled and twisted vessels are interspersed (Fig. 6.8e).

Biological Marker Evidence

In order to provide more evidence to support the presence of angiogenic and lymphangiogenic processes occurring in the lesional skin of Tg mice, we next examined some relevant biological markers.

Tissue and Serum Angiogenic and Lymphangiogenic Factors

VEGF-A, a major promoter of angiogenesis, has been shown to stimulate endothelial cells proliferation, migration, blood vessel sprouting and remodeling. [41] Skin VEGF-A mRNA level and serum VEGF-A protein concentration are increased in IL-4 Tg mice that have developed skin lesions, but not in those that are disease free. Both parameters are higher in Tg mice with chronic skin lesions than early skin lesions, further suggesting that dermal angiogenic stimulation may be closely intertwined with disease progression [38].

While we documented an increase in then total skin VEGF-A mRNA, each of the three VEGF-A isoforms (VEGF-A120, VEGF-A164 and VEGF-A188) was found to have variable expressions in the Tg mice [38]. VEGF-A188 mRNA levels are significantly increased in all disease stages, whereas VEGF-A120 mRNA levels are only increased in lesional skin, but not before disease onset. Interestingly there is no change in VEGF-A164 mRNA level in Tg mice when compared to NT. It is unclear why isoforms 188 and 120 are preferentially over-expressed in the skin of the Tg mice. Since the degree of angiogenesis increases with severity and VEGF-A120 expressions are only increased in lesional skin but not before disease onset, it is possible that VEGF-A120 plays role mainly in the maintenance of inflammatory angiogenesis, but not in its initiation. However, VEGF-A188 isoform is upregulated in all disease stages, suggesting that it may play a role in both the initiation and maintenance stages of skin inflammation. In addition of VEGF-A, the role of a number of other angiogenic factors has been studied in the Tg mice. Their mRNA regulation in various AD disease stages has summarized in Table 6.2.

Conflicting evidence exist regarding the role of various inflammatory cytokines in angiogenesis. Some studies suggest that TNF-alpha and IL1b, but not IL-6 induced VEGF-A mRNA expression in human keratinocytes. [42] Others have shown the opposite findings. [43, 44] In the IL-4 Tg mice, skin IL-6 mRNA expression was elevated in both EL and LL stages compared to NT and BO stages while INF-gamma mRNA was elevated in only LL stage. No change in either cytokine's mRNA levels was seen in the BO stage. Co-stimulation with INF-gamma and IL-6, but not INF-alpha and IL-1β, leads to increased VEGF-A120 mRNA and total VEGF-A protein levels in primary keratinocytes extracted from both NT and Tg mice. The stimulatory role of IL-6 and INF-gamma in angiogenesis was confirmed when intradermal administration of recombinant murine IL-6 and INF-gamma induced VEGF-A120 mRNA elevation in the skin of Tg mice when compared to administration of PBS. [38] So in our study, data supports a role of IL-6 and INF-gamma in angiogenesis.

Real-Time PCR Data

Consistent with immunoflourescence microscope study, the skin mRNA level of VEGFR-2 is significantly increased in acute and chronic lesions of the IL-4 Tg mice. Other pro-angiogenic factors that show mRNA upregulation include Ang-1 and VE-Cadherin. For lymphangiogenesis, markers/factors that show mRNA upregulation in acute and chronic lesions of the IL-4 Tg mice include PDPN, Lyve-1, VEGF-C, Ang-1 and Ang-2. Since Ang-1, Ang-2, and VEGF-C are involved in both

Table 6.2 Change in the mRNA and protein expressions of various angiogenic and lymphangiogenic markers in different disease stages in the K-14-IL Tg mouse

Angiogenesis	Total VEGF-A	VEGF-A120	VEGF-A164	VEGF-A188	VEGF-B	VEGF-C	VEGF-D	VEGFR-1	VEGFR-2	VEGFR-3	VE-Cadherin	Ang-1	Tie-2
mRNA	EL, LL	EL, LL	No change	BO, EL, LL	No change	No change	No change	No change	EL, LL	No change	EL, LL	EL, LL	No change
Protein	EL, LL												

Lymphangiogenesis	PDPN	Lyve-1	VEGFR-3	VEGF-C	VEGF-D	Ang-1	Ang-2
mRNA	BO, EL, LL	BO, EL, LL	BO, EL, LL	EL, LL	No change	EL, LL	BO, EL, LL
Protein	BO, EL, LL	BO, EL, LL	BO, EL, LL				

Data from Chen et al. [38] and Shi et al. [40]

angiogenesis and lymphangiogenesis, it is not clear whether their upreguations favor one process or the other. The mRNA expressions of these factors in different disease stages are summarized in Table 6.2.

Cellular Source of Lymphangiogenic Growth Factor

Many cellular candidates have been proposed as the potential source of hemangiogenic and lymphangiogenic factors in AD. We found that our IL4-Tg mice had augmented dermal infiltration of T cell, mast cell, macrophage-like mononuclear cells, and eosinophils, however the exact contributory role of these inflammatory cells in microvasculature remains elusive. Mast cells may be one cell source for both angiogenesis and lymphangiogenesis due to their intrinsic capacity to produce vascular growth factors (VEGF-A, B, C, and D) and vascular growth factor receptors (VEGFR-1 and 2), their residence in close proximity of blood endothelial cells [30] and their presence at sites of angiogenesis. However, recent data increasingly supports an important role of macrophages in lymphangiogenesis. Activated CD11b+ macrophages express lymphangiogenic markers such as VEGFR-3, VEGF-C, Lyve-1 PDPN and can aggregate to form vessel like-structures in vitro. [45] Primary macrophages express hemangiogenic factors VEGF-A and VEGF-B, and lymphangiogenic factors VEGF-C and D. [46]

We therefore focused our investigation on the role of macrophages in our model. During the course of disease in the IL-4 Tg mouse, there is progressive dermal infiltration of CD11b+ macrophages that exhibit cytoplasmic and peri-cellular VEGF-C immune-reactivity [40] (Fig. 6.9). In support of this hypothetical mechanism, our in vitro experiment showed that IL-4 induced epidermal cells to express macrophage-chemotactic protein (MCP-1) in a dose dependent manner. [40] Taken together, IL-4 may spark local recruitment and trans-differentiation of macrophages into VEGF-C producing cells that drive lymphangiogenesis in AD. In addition, VEGF-C immunoreactivity is absent in the epidermis of the IL-4 Tg mice, ruling out that keratinocytes (and stromal cells) as the major contributor of VEGF-C in the AD mouse model.

Functional Evidence

Increased microvascular permeability is a hallmark of angiogenesis. In addition to vessel enlargement and sprouting, the influence of VEGF on endothelial VEGF receptors has been shown to increased blood vessel leakiness. VEGF administration can induce fenestration development from a continuous endothelium. The analysis of dermal vascular physiology was made possible using Evans blue (EB), a blue colored azo dye with very high affinity for serum albumin, and thus is useful to visualize the functional integrity of blood and lymphatic flow. When EB was injected intravenously into the tail vein of the Tg mice, the ears became dramatically more blue in color in just 5 min when compared to NT [38] (Fig. 6.10). The color intensity and relative EB concentration was significantly greater in the ears of lesional skin (Tg-EL and Tg-LL) than nonlesional skin (Tg-BO). The up-regulation of VEGF-A and VEGFR-2 protein level in all Tg disease stages corroborates morphologic changes of angiogenesis (as illustrated by EM findings), functional

CD11b   VEGF-C   MERGED

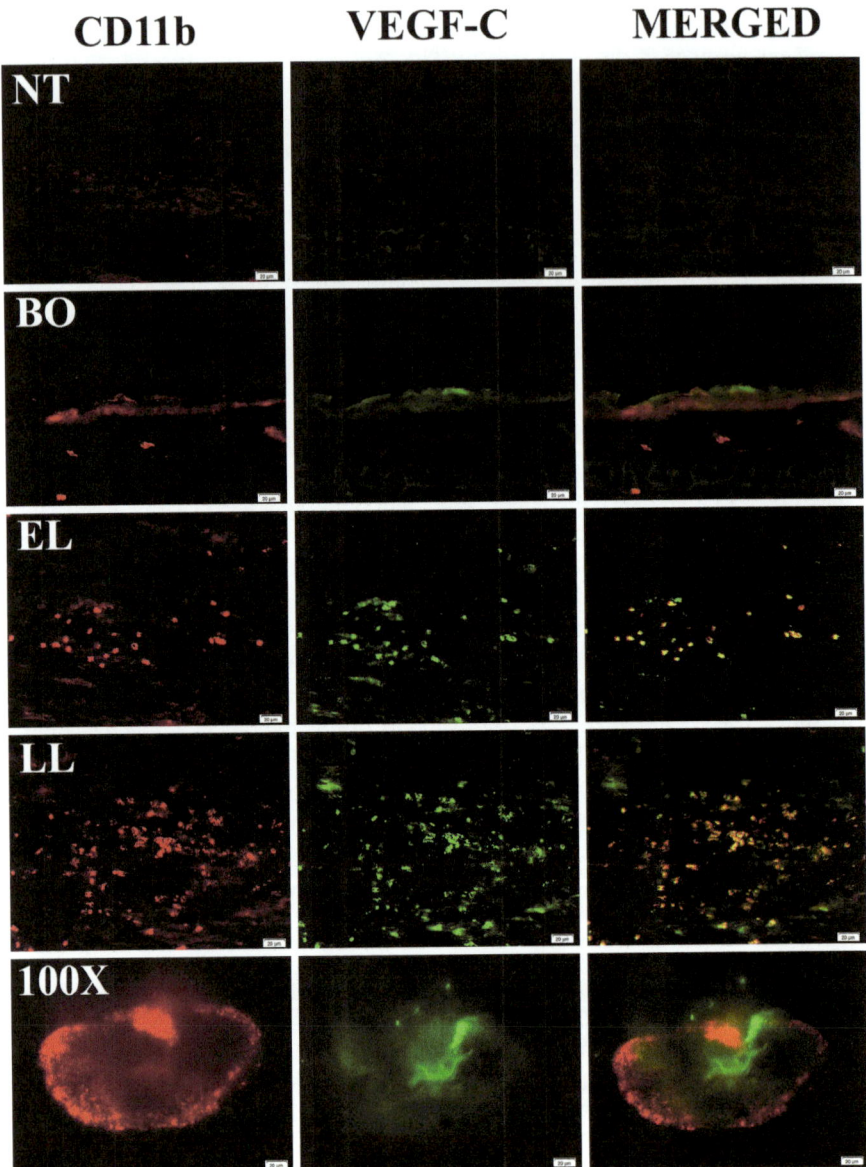

Fig. 6.9 CD11b+ macrophages express VEGF-C in the skin of IL-4 Tg mouse. CD11b+ (*red*) and VEGF-C (*green*) immunoreactivity co-localize in the dermis (merged), their expressions increases with AD severity. VEGF-C expression is seen both intracellular and pericellular of CD11b+ cells (100×, bottom panel) (Reproduced with permission, Shi et al. [40])

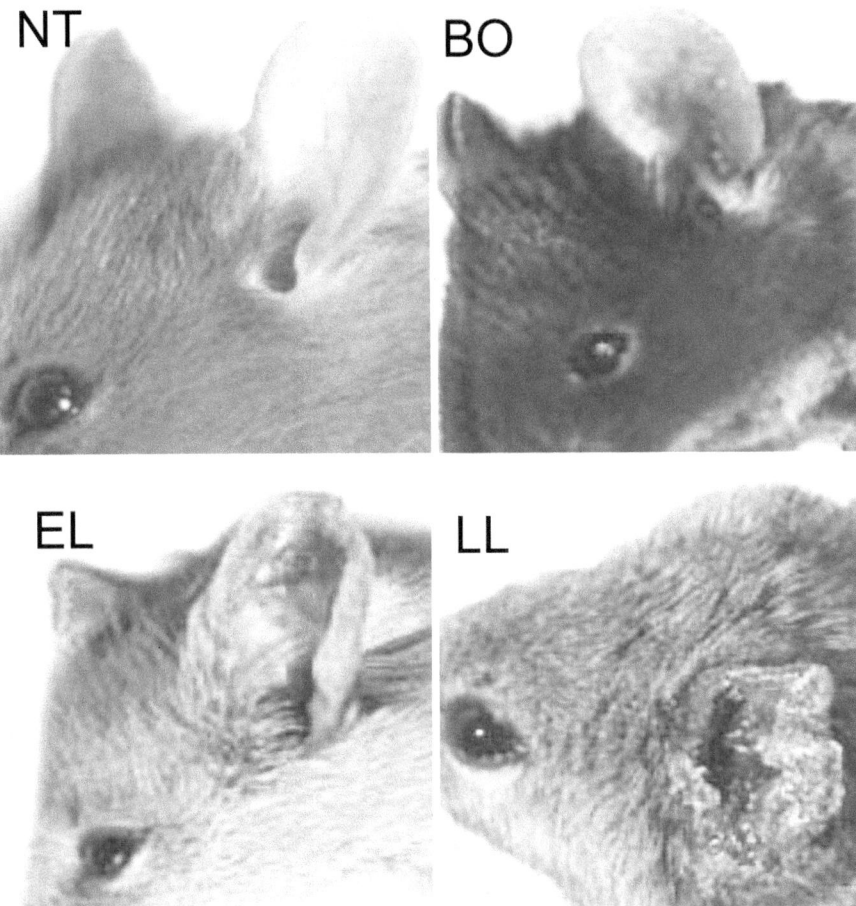

Fig. 6.10 Dermal vascular leakage increases as AD progresses in Tg mice. The vascular leakage is demonstrated by the increasing intensity in the ears of the K-14-IL4 Tg mouse as the disease stages advanced from BO to EL and to LL. (Reproduced with permission, Chen et al. [38])

changes of angiogenesis (as demonstrated by increased microvascular permeability), and inflammation (as depicted by increased inflammatory cell infiltration).

One of the main functions of the lymphatic system is to uptake extravascular fluid and plasma proteins in the interstitial fluid and return them back to the blood stream. We thus examined whether the enlarged and newly formed dermal lymphatic vessels in the IL-4 Tg mice retain their innate functional capacity for active macromolecule uptake. We found that EB was indeed specifically taken up by lymphatic vessels. Twenty-four hours after intradermally administration of EB, the ears of the Tg mice appears lighter in blue color when compared to NT mice (Fig. 6.11) [40]. When we analyzed the extracted dye, we found that the color intensity and relative EB concentration remained in the tissue was inversely proportional to

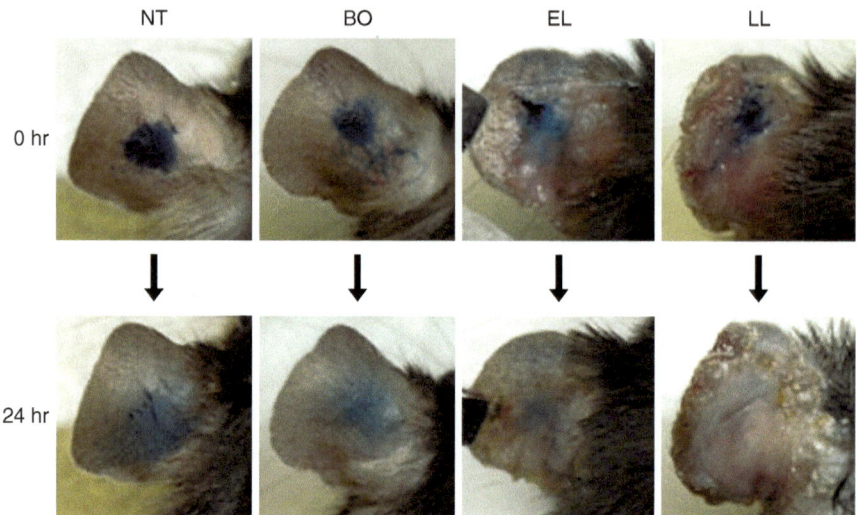

Fig. 6.11 Lymphatic drainage in the ears of the K-14-IL4 Tg mouse increases with AD severity. Dermal lymphatic update is inversely proportional to the amount of dye remaining at 24 h post-injection (Reproduced with permission, Shi et al. [40])

disease severity, indicating lymphangiogenesis associated with skin inflammation retains its native functional integrity, i.e., the new formed lymphatic vessels are capable of up taking fluid.

In Vitro Functional Studies

cDNA Microarray Data

Inflammation-mediated angiogenesis and lymphangiogenesis are likely resulted from of an interplay of cytokines, adhesion molecules, and other factors. Microarray gene study is a useful screening tool for identifying key mediators of angiogenesis and lymphangiogenesis, because it allows accurate assessment of the entire signature within a single experimental process. Since IL-4 is an important initiation of inflammatory process in AD, we investigate how IL-4 might contribute to the angiogenesis and lymphangiogenesis processes through influencing epidermal cells. Indeed we found that IL-4 is a stimulator of VEGF-A up-regulation in human keratinocytes. [31] PCR gene array on inflammation/autoimmunity revealed that 24 h following IL-4 challenge, VEGF-A gene expressions in HaCAT cells were increased 2.2 folds at 10 ng/ml of IL-4, 1.89 folds at 20 ng/ml of IL-4 and 2.73 folds at 50 ng/ml of IL-4. Moreover, IL-4 treatment down regulates TNF superfamily 15, an inhibitor of angiogenesis, in a dose-dependent manner.

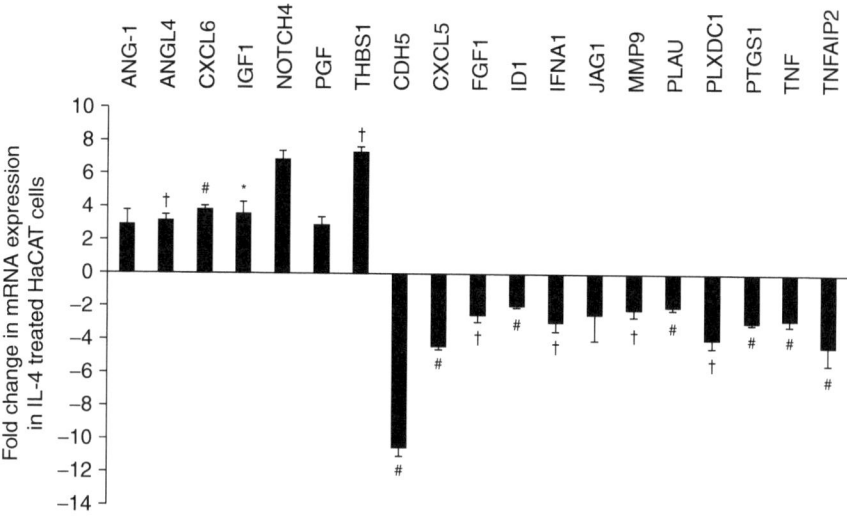

Fig. 6.12 IL-4 regulates the expressions of lymphangiogenic-related genes in human keratinocytes. Upward bars represent up-regulation, downward bars represent down-regulation. *p < 0.05, p < 0.01, #p < 0.001 statistical significance vs. treatment with control (albumin) (Reproduced with permission, Shi et al. [40])

IL-4 stimulation also modulates the expression of a large number of lymphangiogenic-related genes in human keratinocytes. Among these genes, ones that showed over two-fold up- or down-regulations are summarized in (Fig. 6.12). Most of the data on these lymphangiogenic markers thus far have focused on their role in lymphatic metastasis of cancer, their detailed role and mechanism in skin inflammatory diseases has not yet been elucidated. Significantly, IL-4 treatment down-regulates the inhibitors of lymphangiogenesis (INFA1 and TNF). [40] Together, our in vitro data showed that IL-4 not only up-regulates pro-angiogenic and lymphangiogenic factors, but also down-regulates inhibitors of angiogensis and lymphangiogenesis, thus may be a major factor in promoting angiogenesis and lymphangiogenesis.

Summary

Cumulated evidence from human studies allows us to construct a proposed mechanism in which angiogenesis plays a role in the inflammatory process of AD (Fig. 6.13). Up-regualtion of cutaneous inflammatory milieu in human AD including the increase and release of various cytokines and chemokines which lead to recruitment of mast cells and eosinophils into the dermis area. The subsequent release of VEGF-A and VEGF-B by mast cells/eosinophils will lead to their binding to the

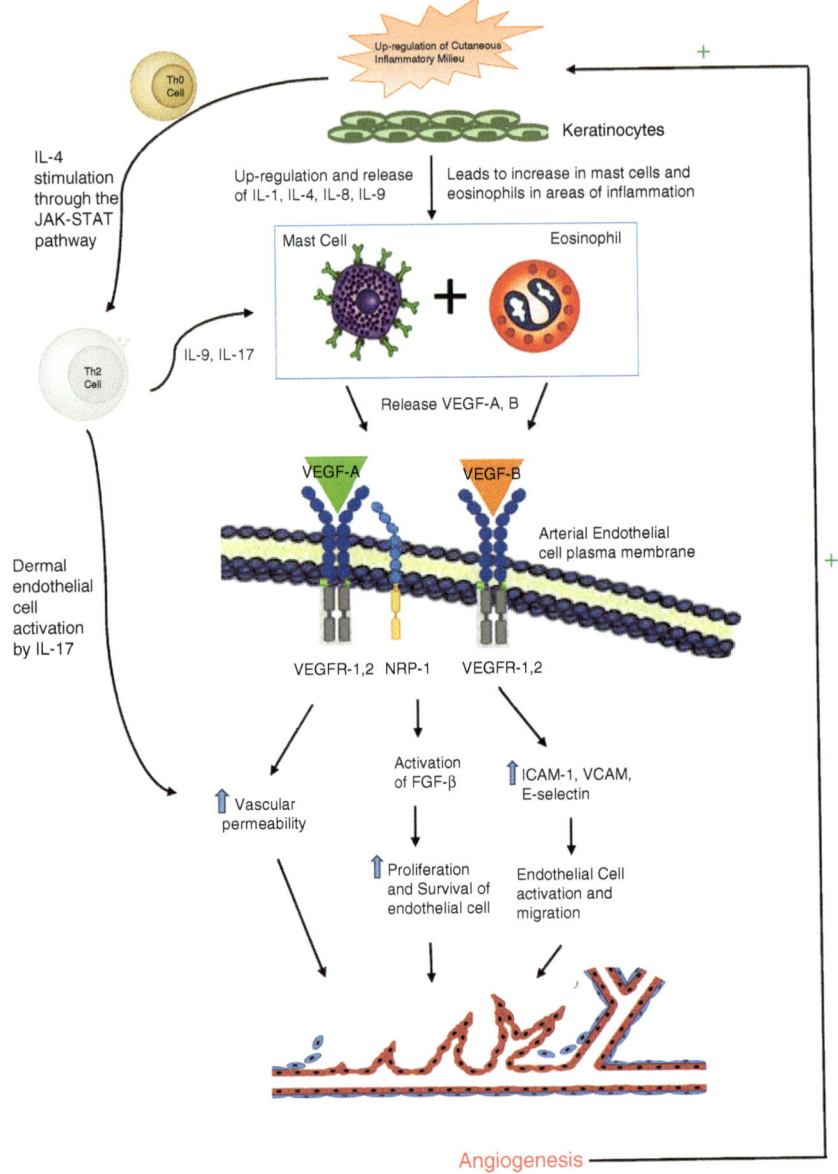

Fig. 6.13 Schematic diagram of the proposed role of angiogenesis in human atopic dermatitis. *Black arrows* indicate direction of influence and/or activation

corresponding endothelial cell receptors VEGFR1, VEGFR2, and NRP-1, resulting in increased vascular permeability, increased proliferation and survival of endothelial cells via FGF-β activation, and endothelial cell activation and migration via up-regulation of ICAM-1, VCAM, and E-selectin, thus promoting microvascular angiogenesis. The vascular permeability is further enhanced by the presence of IL-17 released by activated Th2 cells through IL-4/JAK-STAT signaling pathway. The resulting angiogenesis, moreover, becomes a positive feedback force to enhance and maintain the inflammatory process by providing additional delivery system for the fuel of inflammation. Similarly, data collected from studying the IL-4-Tg mouse model enables us to propose how hymphangiogenesis may contribute to the anti-inflammatory process in AD (Fig. 6.14). Epidermal over-expression of IL-4 initiates an up-regulated cutaneous inflammatory milieu. Particularly, IL-4 stimulates keratinocytes to express MCP-1, which serve as a chemokine to recruit CD11b+ macrophages to the site of skin inflammation. Additionally, IL-4 can cause skin barrier disruption by decreasing synthesis of various barrier proteins (filaggrin, involucine, loricrine). The breakdown of the protective barrier layer enhances bacterial colonization and penetration into the epidermis and dermis. Bacterial components such as lipopolysaccharide (LPS) and lipoteichoic acid (LTA) can induce dermal macrophages to release VEGF-C, which could then stimulate dermal lymphangiogenesis through the binding of its corresponding endothelial cell receptor (VEGFR3). This mechanism is thought to be an attempt to resolve inflammation by clearing inflammatory macromolecules and cells.

Future Research Direction

Existing experimental data thus far strongly suggests that both angiogenesis and lymphangiogenesis play a role in the inflammatory process of AD. While angiogenesis in AD promotes the inflammatory process by providing additional vessels for the delivery of inflammatory cells and mediators to the inflamed site, the lymphangiogenesis in AD seems to act in down-regulating the inflammatory process by providing pathways to remove the inflammatory cells and mediators from the inflamed site. To confirm these biological actions in a functional manner, we need to investigate the in vivo outcomes of both angiogenic inhibitor and lymphangiogenic inhibitor, as our next steps. A logical way would be to examine whether these inhibitors would reverse, make worse, or render no change in the skin inflammation in an animal model of human disease. Should an inhibitor prove to be useful in reversing the inflammatory process in the animal model, it may pave the way for the development of new therapeutic modalities for this chronic inflammatory skin disease.

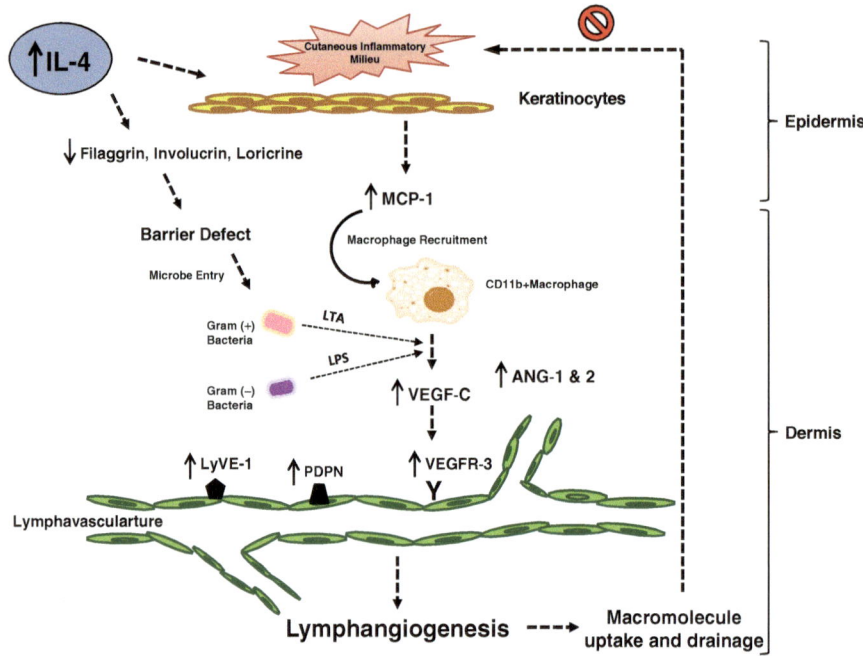

Fig. 6.14 The proposed mechanism of Inflammation-mediated lymphangiogenesis in K14-IL-4 Tg mice model of AD. *Dotted arrows* represent direction of influence. *Solid arrows* represent up- or down-regulation of expression

References

1. Chan LS. Atopic dermatitis in 2008. Curr Dir Autoimmun. 2008;10:76–118.
2. Department of Health. Handout on health: atopic dermatitis. [Homepage on the Internet]. c2011 [updated 2011, August]. Available from http://www.niams.nih.gov/Health_Info/Atopic_Dermatitis/default.asp.
3. Eichenfield LF, Hanifin JM, Beck LA, et al. Atopic dermatitis and asthma: parallels in the evolution of treatment. Pediatrics. 2003;111:608–16.
4. Spergel JM, Paller AS. Atopic dermatitis and the atopic march. J Allergy Clin Immunol. 2003;112:S118–27.
5. Guttman-Yassky E, Nograles KE, Krueger JG. Contrasting pathogenesis of atopic dermatitis and psoriasis–part II: immune cell subsets and therapeutic concepts. J Allergy Clin Immunol. 2011;127:1420–32.
6. Guttman-Yassky E, Nograles KE, Krueger JG. Contrasting pathogenesis of atopic dermatitis and psoriasis–part I: clinical and pathologic concepts. J Allergy Clin Immunol. 2011;127:1110–8.
7. Chen L, Martinez O, Overbergh L, et al. Early up-regulation of Th2 cytokines and late surge of Th1 cytokines in an atopic dermatitis model. Clin Exp Immunol. 2004;138:375–87.
8. Szekanecz Z, Koch AE. Mechanisms of disease: angiogenesis in inflammatory diseases. Nat Clin Pract Rheumatol. 2007;3:635–43.
9. Velasco P, Lange-Asschenfeldt B. Dermatological aspects of angiogenesis. Br J Dermatol. 2002;147:841–52.
10. Ala A, Dhillon AP, Hodgson HJ. Role of cell adhesion molecules in leukocyte recruitment in the liver and gut. Int J Exp Pathol. 2003;84:1–16.

11. Wakita H, Sakamoto T, Tokura Y, et al. E-selectin and vascular cell adhesion molecule-1 as critical adhesion molecules for infiltration of T lymphocytes and eosinophils in atopic dermatitis. J Cutan Pathol. 1994;21:33–9.

12. Steinhoff M, Steinhoff A, Homey B, et al. Role of vasculature in atopic dermatitis. J Allergy Clin Immunol. 2006;118:190–7.

13. Gutgesell C, Heise S, Seubert A, et al. Comparison of different activity parameters in atopic dermatitis: correlation with clinical scores. Br J Dermatol. 2002;147:914–9.

14. de Vries IJ, Langeveld-Wildschut EG, van Reijsen FC, et al. Adhesion molecule expression on skin endothelia in atopic dermatitis: effects of TNF-alpha and IL-4. J Allergy Clin Immunol. 1998;102:461–8.

15. Madej A, Reich A, Orda A, et al. Expression of vascular adhesion protein-1 in atopic eczema. Int Arch Allergy Immunol. 2006;139:114–21.

16. Bieber T. Atopic dermatitis: a paradigmatic allergic skin disease. Mediators Inflamm. 2001;10:291–2.

17. Jung K, Imhof BA, Linse R, et al. Adhesion molecules in atopic dermatitis: upregulation of alpha6 integrin expression in spontaneous lesional skin as well as in atopen, antigen and irritative induced patch test reactions. Int Arch Allergy Immunol. 1997;113:495–504.

18. Jung K, Linse F, Heller R, et al. Adhesion molecules in atopic dermatitis: VCAM-1 and ICAM-1 expression is increased in healthy-appearing skin. Allergy. 1996;51:452–60.

19. Folkman J. Angiogenesis in cancer, vascular, rheumatoid and other disease. Nat Med. 1995;1:27–31.

20. Genovese A, Detoraki A, Granata F, et al. Angiogenesis, lymphangiogenesis and atopic dermatitis. Chem Immunol Allergy. 2012;96:50–60.

21. Carmeliet P, Jain RK. Molecular mechanisms and clinical applications of angiogenesis. Nature. 2011;473:298–307.

22. Gluzman-Poltorak Z, Cohen T, Herzog Y, et al. Neuropilin-2 is a receptor for the vascular endothelial growth factor (VEGF) forms VEGF-145 and VEGF-165 [corrected]. J Biol Chem. 2000;275:18040–5.

23. Soker S, Takashima S, Miao HQ, et al. Neuropilin-1 is expressed by endothelial and tumor cells as an isoform-specific receptor for vascular endothelial growth factor. Cell. 1998;92:735–45.

24. Herzog Y, Kalcheim C, Kahane N, et al. Differential expression of neuropilin-1 and neuropilin-2 in arteries and veins. Mech Dev. 2001;109:115–9.

25. Amarbayasgalan T, Takahashi H, Dekio I, et al. Content of vascular endothelial growth factor in stratum corneum well correlates to local severity of acute inflammation in patients with atopic dermatitis. Int Arch Allergy Immunol. 2012;157:251–8.

26. Kay AB. Calcitonin gene-related peptide- and vascular endothelial growth factor-positive inflammatory cells in late-phase allergic skin reactions in atopic subjects. J Allergy Clin Immunol. 2011;127:232–7.

27. Shahbazi M, Fryer AA, Pravica V, et al. Vascular endothelial growth factor gene polymorphisms are associated with acute renal allograft rejection. J Am Soc Nephrol. 2002;13:260–4.

28. Detoraki A, Staiano RI, Granata F, et al. Vascular endothelial growth factors synthesized by human lung mast cells exert angiogenic effects. J Allergy Clin Immunol. 2009;123:1142–9. 9 e1-5.

29. Steinhoff M, Neisius U, Ikoma A, et al. Proteinase-activated receptor-2 mediates itch: a novel pathway for pruritus in human skin. J Neurosci. 2003;23:6176–80.

30. Groneberg DA, Bester C, Grutzkau A, et al. Mast cells and vasculature in atopic dermatitis–potential stimulus of neoangiogenesis. Allergy. 2005;60:90–7.

31. Bao L, Shi VY, Chan LS. IL-4 up-regulates epidermal chemotactic, angiogenic, and pro-inflammatory genes and down-regulates antimicrobial genes in vivo and in vitro: relevant in the pathogenesis of atopic dermatitis. Cytokine. 2013;61:419–25.

32. Takahashi H, Numasaki M, Lotze MT, et al. Interleukin-17 enhances bFGF-, HGF- and VEGF-induced growth of vascular endothelial cells. Immunol Lett. 2005;98:189–93.

33. Sismanopoulos N, Delivanis DA, Alysandratos KD, et al. IL-9 induces VEGF secretion from human mast cells and IL-9/IL-9 receptor genes are overexpressed in atopic dermatitis. PLoS One. 2012;7:e33271.

34. Homey B, Steinhoff M, Ruzicka T, et al. Cytokines and chemokines orchestrate atopic skin inflammation. J Allergy Clin Immunol. 2006;118:178–89.

35. Chan LS, Robinson N, Xu L. Expression of interleukin-4 in the epidermis of transgenic mice results in a pruritic inflammatory skin disease: an experimental animal model to study atopic dermatitis. J Invest Dermatol. 2001;117:977–83.

36. Hanifin JM, Rajka G. Diagnostic features of atopic dermatitis. Acta Derm Venereol Suppl (Stockh). 1980;92:4.

37. Henno A, Blacher S, Lambert CA, et al. Histological and transcriptional study of angiogenesis and lymphangiogenesis in uninvolved skin, acute pinpoint lesions and established psoriasis plaques: an approach of vascular development chronology in psoriasis. J Dermatol Sci. 2010;57:162–9.

38. Chen L, Marble DJ, Agha R, et al. The progression of inflammation parallels the dermal angiogenesis in a keratin 14 IL-4-transgenic model of atopic dermatitis. Microcirculation. 2008;15:49–64.

39. Agha-Majzoub R, Becker RP, Schraufnagel DE, et al. Angiogenesis: the major abnormality of the keratin-14 IL-4 transgenic mouse model of atopic dermatitis. Microcirculation. 2005;12:455–76.

40. Shi VY, Bao L, Chan LS. Inflammation-Driven Dermal Lymphangiogenesis in Atopic Dermatitis is Associated with CD11b+ Macrophage Recruitment and VEGF-C Up-regulation in the IL-4-Transgenic Mouse Model. Microcirculation. 2012;19:567–79.

41. Stephan CC, Brock TA. Vascular endothelial growth factor, a multifunctional polypeptide. P R Health Sci J. 1996;15:169–78.

42. Frank S, Hubner G, Breier G, et al. Regulation of vascular endothelial growth factor expression in cultured keratinocytes. Implications for normal and impaired wound healing. J Biol Chem. 1995;270:12607–13.

43. Trompezinski S, Denis A, Vinche A, et al. IL-4 and interferon-gamma differentially modulate vascular endothelial growth factor release from normal human keratinocytes and fibroblasts. Exp Dermatol. 2002;11:224–31.

44. Detmar M, Yeo KT, Nagy JA, et al. Keratinocyte-derived vascular permeability factor (vascular endothelial growth factor) is a potent mitogen for dermal microvascular endothelial cells. J Invest Dermatol. 1995;105:44–50.

45. Maruyama K, Ii M, Cursiefen C, et al. Inflammation-induced lymphangiogenesis in the cornea arises from CD11b-positive macrophages. J Clin Invest. 2005;115:2363–72.

46. Granata F, Frattini A, Loffredo S, et al. Production of vascular endothelial growth factors from human lung macrophages induced by group IIA and group X secreted phospholipases A2. J Immunol. 2010;184:5232–41.

Chemoprevention and Angiogenesis

7

Shikha Rao, Rebecca A. Pankove, Jiaqi Mi, Justin Elsey, and Jack L. Arbiser

Introduction

An estimated one in five Americans will develop skin cancer in their lifetime [1]. In 2016, melanoma is estimated to account for approximately 5% (76380) of all expected new cancer cases by the American cancer society and with estimated death of 10130 people due to the disease [2]. Men have a 3% chance of developing invasive melanoma, amounting to 1 in 33 men in the US while women have a 1.9% chance equating to 1 in 52 women in the US [2]. In addition, non-melanoma skin cancers, including basal and squamous cell carcinoma represent the most common of cancers, with over 1 million new cases per year [3]. However, these statistics are likely an underestimate due to underreporting. Fortunately, for those whose melanoma is detected and treated before it spreads to the lymph nodes, the five-year survival rate is 98%. On the other hand, the five-year survival rate for distant stage

S. Rao
Department of Dermatology, Emory University School of Medicine, Atlanta, GA, USA
e-mail: srao30@emory.edu

R.A. Pankove
Department of Dermatology, Emory University School of Medicine, Atlanta, GA, USA
e-mail: rpankov@emory.edu

J. Mi
Medical College of Georgia, Augusta, GA, USA
e-mail: JMI@augusta.edu

J. Elsey
Department of Dermatology, Emory University School of Medicine, Atlanta, GA, USA
e-mail: justin.elsey@emory.edu

J.L. Arbiser (✉)
Department of Dermatology, Emory University School of Medicine and Atlanta VA Medical Center, Atlanta, GA, USA
e-mail: jarbise@emory.edu

© Springer-Verlag London Ltd. 2017
J.L. Arbiser (ed.), *Angiogenesis-Based Dermatology*,
DOI 10.1007/978-1-4471-7314-4_7

melanomas is 17%, a mortality rate second only to lung cancer and continues to rise due to increased sun exposure, and environmental carcinogens, despite increased public awareness [4, 5].

Populations especially susceptible to the damaging effects of UVA and UVB rays and developing skin cancer are those who spend extended periods of time in the sun or in tanning beds over a lifetime, those who have had at least one severe sunburn, those with a family history or inherited disorder, people with fair skin, light hair, and light eyes, people with dysplastic nevi, and those who suffer from certain skin disorders such as actinic keratosis and Human Papilloma Virus (HPV) [6]. Chronic exposure to UV rays can also have less severe consequences such as photoaging. Photoaging is a type of damage characterized by histological changes in the dermal connective tissues such as damage to collagen fibers, excessive deposition of abnormal elastic fibers, and increased levels of glycosaminoglycans [7]. The result of these changes is a wrinkled, lax and coarse appearance along with brown spots and uneven pigmentation [8].

Skin tumor formation has three stages: tumor initiation, tumor promotion, and tumor progression (Fig. 7.1). UVA (315–400nm) and UVB (280-315nm) rays from the sun are related to 70% of melanoma cases and are considered complete carcinogens: they can both initiate and promote cancer [9–11]. UVA, the largest portion of solar radiation reaching the earth acts as a tumor promoter while UVB is 1000–10,000 times more carcinogenic per J/m2 than UVA and functions as a tumor initiator [8, 12]. Their role in skin cancer is multifaceted, causing chromosomal alternations and DNA damage either directly or indirectly through reactive oxygen species (ROS) [8, 13]. UVB causes direct DNA damage, creating cyclobutane dimers, photoproducts, cytosine photohydrates, DNA strand breaks, and crosslinks, damage that cannot be reverted by nucleotide excision repair. UVA does not directly affect DNA, but rather induces oxidative damage by generating ROS [10]. When UVA contacts the skin, endogenous photosensitizers such as porphyrins and NADH become excited and react with oxygen to create hydrogen peroxide and hydroxyl radicals that cause miscoding lesions in DNA. These ROS are also capable of stimulating tumor development independent of DNA damage, by lipid peroxidation of the cell membrane and subsequent activation of signaling pathways such as those that regulate the proinflammatory transcription factor NF-kB [8]. High levels of reactive oxygen also induce DNA methyl transferase 1 (DNMT), which methylates tumor suppressors such as p16ink4a. This is part of the generation of the reactive oxygen induced tumor, which uses Akt and reactive oxygen for oncogenic signaling [14]. This increase in inflammation also has a strong relationship with skin aging, as the combination of ROS over-generation and aging as the immune system becomes less able to manage an inflammatory response [13].

This ROS induced irreversible DNA damage can induce vascular changes, through recruitment of cytokines and chemokines such as vascular endothelial growth factor (VEGF), basic fibroblast growth factor (b-FGF) and interleukin-8 (IL-8) [15]. These discernable and internal changes can further upregulate oncogenic and inflammatory pathways associated with skin cancer including MAPK, EGFR, Src, and p53 mutations [16]. In addition, it can further affect skin

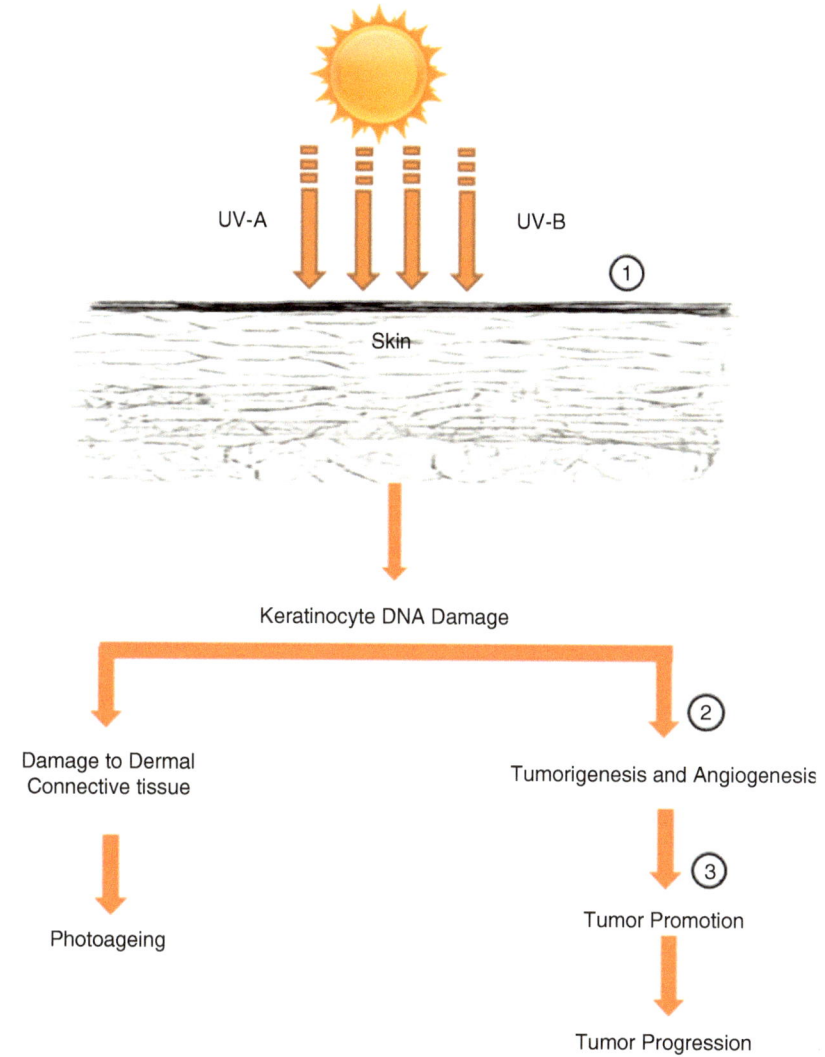

Fig. 7.1 Cancer transformation is a multi-stage process and chemopreventive strategies should aim to target the exposure (1), and/or initial cancer formation (2) or (3) cancer promotion

appearance, causing erythema, epidermal hyperplasia, vascular dilation and hyper-permeability [17].

Aside from excessive sunlight, people are continuously exposed exogenously whether through food, air, or water to chemical carcinogens and mutagens. Chemical carcinogens are hypothesized to contribute to a significant amount of human cancers, particularly through certain foods and tobacco products. Aflatoxin is one such carcinogen found in the diets of Asian and African communities. Aflatoxin is a mold-produced mycotoxin that directly affects the liver and synergizes with hepatitis B virus. Another chemical carcinogen are heterocyclic amines, produced when muscle meats are heated above 180°C for extended time periods. Though of all the ubiquitously present environmental carcinogens, tobacco products are probably the most notorious. Tobacco products contain a host of chemical carcinogens such as polycyclic hydrocarbons, nitrosamines, and aromatic amines which cause the formation of DNA adducts that lead to miscoding and permanent mutations [18].

Because of its high incidence, skin cancer is one of the most pressing issues in cancer today, and has sparked a need to delay the occurrence of cancer in high-risk populations through dietary or chemical interventions [19]. High-risk populations would include solid organ transplant patients on immunosuppressive drugs, patients with DNA repair defects, as well as those with extensive sun exposure, fair skin, and red hair [20, 21]. Patients who are heterozygous for p16ink4a have multiple atypical nevi and a high incidence of melanoma [22]. Cancers such as melanoma have limited treatment options at late stages, are highly metastatic, and develop rapid drug resistance [13].As a result, scientists conduct research on chemoprevention, the use of synthetic or natural agents that inhibit cellular mechanisms involved in tumorigenesis or before invasion and metastasis occur through prevention, arrest, or reversal [23, 24]. Because cancer transformation is a multistage process, three types of chemopreventive strategies exist: those that inhibit initial cancer formation, those that block cancer promotion, and those that prevent recurrence after anti-cancer therapy [25, 26]. Ideal chemopreventive agents must have little toxicity in healthy populations, and distinctly affect premalignant or malignant cells, rendering normal cells unaffected [27]. In order to develop such drugs researchers must know associated pathways, enzymes, genetic alterations, and cellular targets that are critical to cancer development [28].

Of the tumorigenic pathways researched for chemoprevention, angiogenesis, a hallmark of cancer, is one such targeted event. Angiogenesis is the growth of blood vessels with functions in both normal tissues and cancer cells [16]. In normal tissue, angiogenesis is tightly regulated and fundamental to reproduction, development, and tissue repair [29]. In healthy tissues, vasculature is smaller and abundant with evenly spaced, well-differentiated arteries, arterioles, capillaries, venules, and veins [30]. Tumor vasculature, however, is characterized by a large size with some smooth muscle coating, lack of organization, irregular branching, inconsistent blood flow path and leakiness [28, 30]. These characteristics are a result of hypoxia, inflammation, and oncogenic mutations which make healthy tissues undergo an "angiogenic switch" and upregulate pro-angiogenic agents [31]. For a cancer to grow beyond several millimeters and adopt a metastatic phenotype, tumors must have an autonomous blood supply through neovascularization [15]. This abnormal angiogenesis can lead to zones of ischemia and necrosis as the tumor grows and requires more oxygen and nutrients from the blood supply [30].

The balance between angiogenic factors and angiogenic inhibitors can be disrupted by the aforementioned "angiogenic switch." These occurrences can cause the increased secretion of angiogenic factors such as cyclooxygenase-2 (COX-2), a pro-inflammatory enzyme, hypoxia induced factor alpha (HIF-1a) a transcription factor that facilitates response to hypoxia, angiopoetin-1 (ANGPT1), an endothelial cell specific growth factor, angiopoetin-2 (ANGPT2), a vascular endothelium remodeler, matrix metalloproteinases (MMPs), extra-cellular matrix remodelers, and basic/acidic fibroblast growth factor (b-FGF or a-FGF), a growth factor involved in cell mitosis and migration, and local immunologic tolerance among others [16, 30, 32, 33]. BFGF is found to be highly expressed in basal cell carcinoma [34] and mutations in FGFR3 are present in some seborrheic keratosis [35]. Though of the numerous promoters of angiogenesis, vascular endothelial growth factor (VEGF) is perhaps the biggest driver. VEGF is an endothelial cell mitogen that when expressed causes blood vessel growth in both normal and abnormal tissue [36]. Aside from cancer, overexpression of VEGF and persistent angiogenesis supports the progression of certain other inflammatory diseases such as ocular neovascularization, which causes blindness, infantile hemangiomas, arthritis, and psoriasis [37–40].

Though the overexpression of a multitude of angiogenic factors is essential for tumor angiogenesis, the suppression of endogenous angiogenic inhibitors is also necessary for tumorigenesis and metastasis. Such endogenous inhibitors include: angiostatin, involved in cell cycle arrest and apoptosis; endostatin, an inhibitor of cell proliferation and migration; canstatin and tumstatin, inducers of apoptosis; arrestin, an inhibitor of VEGF driven angiogenesis and thromospondin-1 (TSP-1) [15, 29, 33].

NSAIDs and COX-2 Inhibitors

Cyclooxygenase (COX), is the rate-limiting enzyme in the metabolism of arachidonic acid to prostaglandins, and exists in two isoforms: COX-1 and COX-2 [41, 42]. COX-1 is constitutively expressed in bodily tissue while COX-2 is induced by certain pathological processes involving inflammation, mitogens, and growth factors [43]. Cyclooxengenase-2 (COX-2) is a vital enzyme that mediates many inflammatory processes, and whose up-regulation is associated with numerous inflammatory disorders and cancers [44]. Animal models have demonstrated the ability for COX-2 to catalyze malignant transformation [45], and is implicated in human cancers with inflammatory origins such as colorectal, gastric, ovarian, cervical, esophageal, and Non-Melanoma Skin Cancer (NMSC) [46, 47]. Tumor promoters, pro-inflammatory cytokines, lipopolysaccharide (LPS), and growth factors can regulate the expression of COX-2 at the transcriptional and posttranscriptional level. While COX-2 is an essential enzyme in the body, its constitutive expression can initiate and promote carcinogenesis [48]. Some cancer-causing substances that initiate this constitutive expression are chemicals in tobacco smoke such as nicotine, nitrosamines, and poly-cyclic aromatic hydrocarbons [49, 50]. These initiators can also come from the environment, the body, and infectious agents such as some fatty acids [51], radiation [52], ultraviolet B [53], free radicals [54], oncogenic proteins [55], growth factors [56], helicobacter pylori [57], HPV [58], hepatitis viruses [59] and Epstein Barr virus [60]. This continuous over-expression of COX-2 promotes carcinogenesis by mutagenesis through increasing reactive oxygen species, mitogenesis through increased production of prostaglandins, angiogenesis by stimulation of vascular endothelial growth factor (VEGF) and platelet-derived growth factor (PDGF), metastasis by increasing production of matrix metalloproteinases (MMP), anti-apoptosis by decreasing arachidonic acid and inhibition of BAX, immunosuppression through the inhibition of B and T lymphocyte proliferation [61] and heightened intracellular telomerase [62].

Since the 1960's, epidemiological, clinical, and experimental studies have shown the anti-cancer effects of nonsteroidal anti-inflammatory drugs (NSAIDs) through inhibition of COX (Fig. 7.2) [63]. NSAIDs are a family of drugs that are frequently used for inflammation, pain, and fever by reducing the production of specific prostaglandins that promote the aforementioned symptoms along with carcinogenesis [64, 65]. NSAIDs are classified depending on their selective inhibition on the COX isoforms: Selective COX-1 inhibitors, non-selective COX inhibitors, and preferential COX-2 inhibitors [66]. Common NSAIDs like aspirin, ibuprofen, sulindac, and indomethacin inhibit both COX-1 and COX-2 [67] while the later developed coxibs (celecoxib and rofecoxib) selectively inhibit COX-2 [48].

Preclinical studies have shown that NSAIDs such as sulindac sulfide [68], exisulind [69], and celecoxib [70] can inhibit angiogenesis and cell invasion by inhibiting the DNA-binding activity of Sp1, a driver of VEGF overexpression, and by downregulating MMPs [71, 72]. Studies have also shown that Sulindac can stimulate apoptosis in the normal rectal mucosa of patients with familial adenomatous polyposis coli (FAP) [73] by inhibiting Wnt signaling [74] and reducing β-catenin levels [75]. In addition, sulindac, sulindac sulfide, exisulind, and aspirin can inhibit

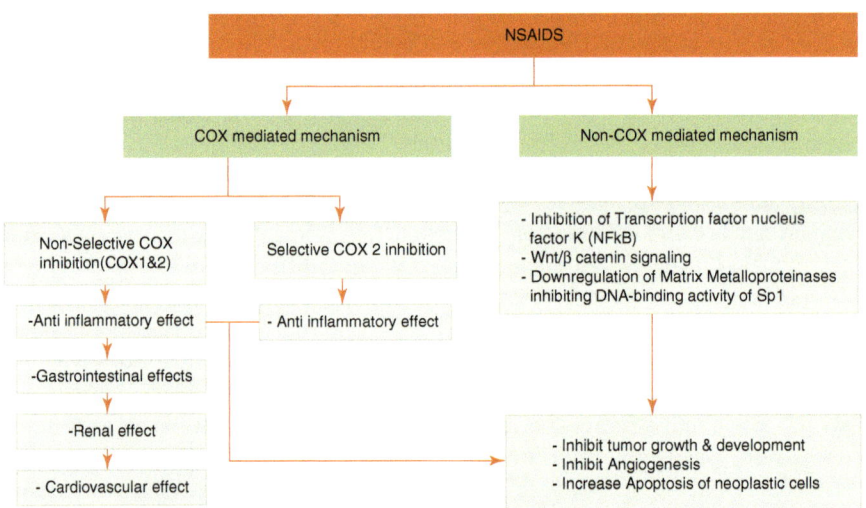

Fig. 7.2 Proposed chemopreventive mechanism of NSAIDS

NF- κB signaling [76, 77]. These agents may also impact the development of NMSC, further proving its efficacy as cancer chemopreventive agents [28].

While COX may be the primary target for NSAIDs, evidently their effect on signaling pathways may also contribute to its chemopreventive properties [24]. Numerous clinical studies have shown the protective effects that NSAIDs have against cancer: Regular intake of 325mg aspirin or 200mg ibuprofen showed a risk reduction of 43% for colon cancer, 25% for breast cancer, 28% for lung cancer, and 27% for prostate cancer [23]. Furthermore, daily intake of selective COX-2 inhibitors, 200mg celecoxib or 25mg rofecoxib, demonstrated a 70% risk reduction in the aforementioned cancers compared to 60% for ibuprofen (COX-1 and COX-2 inhibitor) and 54% for aspirin (COX-1 inhibitor) [23].

However, despite its favorable results, the use of non-selective NSAIDs as a chemopreventive agent is not routinely recommended because of the gastrointestinal and renal side effects that result from the suppression of prostaglandins due to COX inhibition [24]. Therefore, selective inhibition of COX-2 to treat neoplastic proliferation is preferable to non-selective inhibition [78]. By the end of the 90s, the coxib family of drugs was produced to overcome these harsh side effects [79]. Unfortunately, these new drugs caused an increased incidence of cardiovascular side effects after prolonged use [80]. As a result, though clinical studies have shown promising results for using NSAIDs as cancer chemoprevention, long-term administration of COX-2 inhibitors would be ineffective as the risks outweigh the benefits.

Chemoprevention of Basal Cell Nevus Syndrome (BCNS)

BCNS is a rare autosomal dominant disorder characterized by the development of innumerable basal cell carcinomas as well as an increased incidence of medulloblastoma. In addition, other abnormalities are present, including bifid ribs, keratogenic odontocysts, and palmar pits [81].

The major cause of morbidity and mortality in these patients is basal cell carcinoma, which can be locally invasive and rarely metastatic. BCNS is caused by germ line mutations in PTCH, a receptor for the secreted protein Sonic hedgehog. Mutations in PTCH lead to chronic activation of Smoothened and cell proliferation [82]. Smoothened is a transmembrane protein and activator in the Sonic hedgehog pathway [82]. Recently, Smoothened inhibitors have been introduced into the clinic, especially for large and inoperable basal cell carcinomas [83].

These inhibitors shrink but do not completely eliminate large basal cell carcinomas. However, small basal cell carcinomas as in BCNS completely regress. Because these inhibitors can have severe side effects, they are often given intermittently, and thus can be given to patients for long periods of time. It may be possible to use these agents to prevent future development of BCC in patients with BCNS. Azole antifungals have been shown to inhibit this pathway as an off target effect, but small clinical trials have not revealed impressive results [84].

Curcumin

Curcumin (diferuloylmethane) is a yellow phytochemical produced by some plants, especially turmeric (Curcuma longa), a member of the ginger family (Zingiberaceae). Turmeric has been used for thousands of years in Ayurvedic and traditional Chinese medicine due to its antioxidant, anti-inflammatory, anti-tumorigenic, and antiangiogenic properties [85] but has only entered clinical trials in the last 15 years [86].

Curcumin is commonly found as an herbal supplement, an additive in cosmetics, a flavoring agent, and a food coloring. Studies show that turmeric inhibits and decreases the number of tumors in DMBA(7,12-dimethylbenzanthracene) induced and chronic UV initiated and 12-O-tetradecanoylphorbol-13-acetate (TPA) promoted mouse models of chemical carcinogenesis [87, 88]. While many chemotherapeutic agents may severely damage normal cells, curcumin can be safely administered in large quantities with little to no side effects, due to its preference for inducing apoptosis in highly proliferating cells [89]. As a result, curcumin could be a useful dietary additive or pharmacological treatment for the prevention of cancer incidence and mortality.

Curcumin inhibits the activity of interleukins, a group of pro-inflammatory cytokines that play vital roles in the induction of adhesion molecules, metalloproteinases, and pro-angiogenic factors. In addition, interleukins are involved in tumor invasion and angiogenesis through signaling pathways such as NF-kB, VEGF and JAK-STAT, which are inhibited by Curcumin [90–92]. The inhibition of NF-kB plays a central role in general inflammation and immune response. Suppression of COX-2 expression by inhibiting ERK activity and NF-kB activation may represent molecular mechanisms underlying this anti-inflammatory effect [93, 94]. VEGF overexpression, in particular, promotes angiogenesis and tumor growth in a number of cancers including colon, lung, and pancreas. Therefore, agents that inhibit VEGF expression have promising chemotherapeutic potential. In fact, a previous study demonstrated curcumin's ability to inhibit VEGF expression in murine pancreatic and ovarian tumors in a similar action to Avastin (bevacizumab), an FDA-approved drug for certain cancers [95].

In 1998, Arbiser et al showed that Curcumin and its derivatives demonstrated a significant inhibition of bFGF-mediated corneal neovascularization in the mice suggesting that curcumin is a direct angiogenesis inhibitor. Furthermore they also noted effective inhibition of endothelial cell proliferation by Curcumin in a dose-dependent manner [96]. Fibroblast growth factors (FGF) are a family of growth factors involved in angiogenesis and are overexpressed in a variety of tumors.

Curcumin plays a significant role in the abrogation of a number of inflammatory and oncogenic pathways like COX-2 expression (Fig. 7.3). In a study performed in 2005, treatment of UVB-irradiated HaCaT cells with up-regulated COX-2 with curcumin strongly inhibited COX-2 mRNA and protein expression. Notably, there was also effective inhibition on UVB-induced activations of p38, MAPK, AP-1 and JNK. These results collectively suggest that curcumin may be an effective sunscreen for the protection from photo-inflammation [97]. Despite its relatively low toxicity, curcumin has poor bioavailability due to its rapid metabolism in the liver and

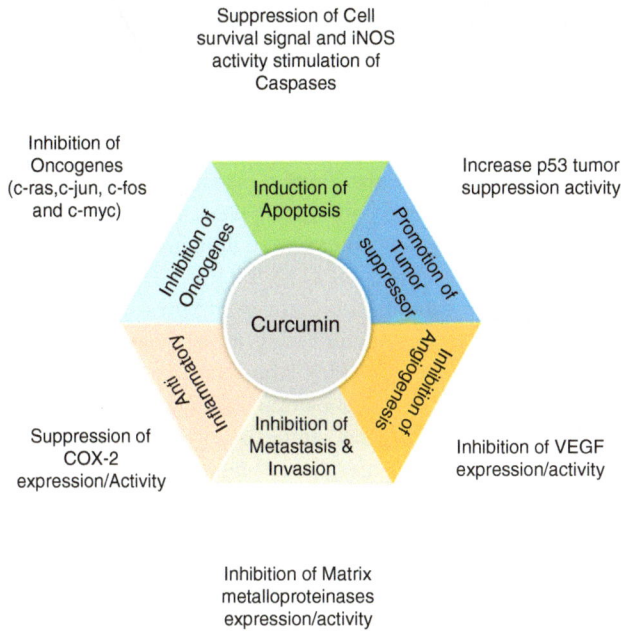

Suppression of Cell survival signal and iNOS activity stimulation of Caspases

Inhibition of Oncogenes (c-ras,c-jun, c-fos and c-myc)

Increase p53 tumor suppression activity

Induction of Apoptosis

Inhibition of Oncogenes

Promotion of Tumor suppressor

Curcumin

Anti Inflammatory

Inhibition of Angiogenesis

Suppression of COX-2 expression/Activity

Inhibition of Metastasis & Invasion

Inhibition of VEGF expression/activity

Inhibition of Matrix metalloproteinases expression/activity

Fig. 7.3 Chemopreventive effects of Curcumin as suggested in human/ animal studies

intestinal tract [98]. As a result, until scientists can develop a method for increasing the bioavailability of curcumin, it may not be an effective chemopreventive method despite its obvious benefits.

Long-chain n-3 Polyunsaturated Fatty Acids

Long-chain n-3 polyunsaturated fatty acids (LC n-3 PUFAs), also known as Omega-3 fatty acids, are essential for normal metabolism [99]. The three types of LC n-3 PUFAs involved in human health are eicosapentaenoic acid (EPA) and docosahexaenoic acid (DHA), which have protective effects on the heart, and alpha-linoleic acid (ALA). LC n-3 PUFAs are not naturally produced in the body, and thus must be obtained through the diet. EPA and DHA are commonly found in marine oils such as fish and krill, while ALA is found in plant oils such as flaxseed, chia, and hemp. Because LC n-3 PUFAs have anti-inflammatory, antiangiogenic, and anticancer properties, their beneficial effects against cancers are widely documented [100, 101]. Numerous clinical studies support the role of n-3 PUFAs for the prevention of both melanoma and non-melanoma skin cancer (NMSC) and primarily attributes their activity to EPA and DHA [101, 102]. In addition to being an effective chemopreventive agent, studies have shown that nutritionally induced changes in tumor fatty acid composition result in increased sensitivity to chemotherapy. This effect is especially observed in chemotherapy resistant tumor lines, by causing augmented cytotoxicity to tumor cells while protecting normal cells [103].

Preclinical studies on LC n-3 PUFAs demonstrate its strong antineoplastic, apoptotic, anti-metastatic, and antiangiogenic activities due to the number of molecular factors and pathways affected. Laboratory experiments show the ability of DHA to prevent UV-induced apoptosis by increasing the expression of the anti-apoptotic Bcl-2 protein, and inhibiting the expression of human antigen R (HuR), which promotes the inflammatory properties of COX-2 [104]. The decreased expression of COX-2 also decreases B-catenin, a protein overexpressed in many cancers [105, 106]. Lastly, DHA has a pro-differentiating effect, which is integral to evade a malignant cell phenotype [105]. Other laboratory experiments demonstrate that EPA can decrease invasiveness, collagenase IV production, and metastasis in melanoma cells [107]. In addition, animal studies show that an omega-3 fatty acid rich diet significantly reduces the growth rate and angiogenesis of a human breast cancer xenograft without evidence of harmful side effects [108].

Recent clinical trials have shown the chemopreventive role of n-23 PUFAs in abrogating photo-immunosuppression [109] and decreasing inflammation [110]. Specifically, -3 PUFAs have shown antitumor activity, while -6 PUFAs and its derived eicosanoids promote anti-carcinogenesis, anti-angiogenesis, and prevent invasion [111]. Administering n-3 PUFAs decreases mucosal and epidermal response, while moderately enhancing the antitumor effect of irradiation. The magnitude of the differential effect suggests that n-3 PUFAs need to be further investigated in the clinic [112].

The mechanism underlying the antineoplastic effect of PUFAs is unclear. Initially, the idea was that n-3 PUFAs have health benefits, and do not produce dangerous levels of cytotoxic and carcinogenic oxidative products in tissues [108]. Another proposed mechanism was that lipid raft signaling proteins can be modulated in inflammation and cancer by n -3 PUFAs [113]. Recent pharmacological studies have suggested several molecular targets for the anti-inflammatory effects of omega-3 fatty acids, namely, nuclear receptor PPARc and the G protein-coupled receptor GPR120. Another proposed mechanism is that omega-3 fatty acids are converted to resolvins and protectins, lipids that have anti-inflammatory and tissue healing activity [114].

Nevertheless, further effort is needed to identify the main molecular targets of LC n-3 PUFAs in melanoma through additional well-designed human observational studies.

Vitamin A

Vitamin A and its analogs represent a group of diverse organic compounds including carotenoids and retinoids, which all have structural or biological effects similar to vitamin A [115]. In the diet, carotenoids are found in leafy green and yellow vegetables, while retinoids exist naturally in the liver and kidneys [116]. Vitamin A and its derivatives regulate a variety of essential biological processes during normal development including vision, cell proliferation and differentiation, bone tissue growth, immune function, and activation of tumor suppressor genes. While Vitamin A is a vital part of a healthy diet, its derivative, retinoids, are important in maintaining skin health and reducing susceptibility to chemical carcinogens [117] by regulating gene expression [118]. The major skin diseases that benefit from treatment with topical retinoids such as tretinoin are acne, psoriasis, disorders of keratinization, premalignant lesions such as actinic keratosis and HPV-induced tumors, and non-melanoma skin cancer [119]. Because of its apparent chemopreventive properties, patients at high risk for skin cancer due to genetic disposition (xeroderma pigmentosum), organ transplantation, or history of multiple tumors, may be treated with retinoids like etretinate or acitretin for 6 months [120].

Retinoids such as etretinate, acitretin, and isotretinoin are most effective in the treatment of precancerous lesions, such as leukoplakias, cervical dysplasia, and actinic keratosis [119]. Tazarotene, a topical retinoid, demonstrated a sustained chemopreventive effect in patients with basal cell nevus syndrome and inhibition of microscopic basal cell carcinomas even 5 months after treatment stopped [121]. These anticancer effects of applied retinoids are attributed to their impact on cellular metabolism, cell cycle progression, and inflammatory pathways. Retinoids upregulate RARβ2 [122], a tumor suppression gene, and induces the expression of p21CIP1 and p27Kip1, cell cycle regulatory proteins that cause growth arrest [123, 124]. Lastly, retinoids effectively modulate inflammatory pathways that are critical for carcinogenesis such as COX-2 [125], IL-6 and HIF-1α [126].

Despite promising *in vitro* and *in vivo* data, some prospective observational studies and randomized controlled trials on retinoids have exhibited a number of side effects. Prolonged exposure to retinoids can cause dry skin, cheilitis, conjunctivitis, and hypertriglyceridemia, effects that can exclude certain individuals from participating. Furthermore, retinoids can be teratogenic, which is a concern for women [127]. The adverse effects demonstrate the importance of finding a retinoid or treatment option that reduces these side effects, as the chemopreventive properties of retinoids are highly promising.

Vitamin D

Vitamin D is a fat-soluble vitamin that is naturally present in very few foods and is available as a dietary supplement. Most commonly, vitamin D is produced endogenously when ultraviolet rays from sunlight strike the skin and trigger vitamin D synthesis. Vitamin D plays a vital role in calcium homeostasis, cell proliferation and cell differentiation [128]. However, the vitamin D obtained from sun exposure, food, and supplements is biologically inert and must be activated inside of the body. The first hydroxylation occurs in the liver, and converts vitamin D to calcidiol (25-hydroxyvitamin D). The second occurs primarily in the kidney, and forms calcitriol (1,25-dihydroxyvitamin D) [129]. This physiologically active calcitriol is then free to bind to the vitamin D receptor (VDR) which affects gene expression by regulating transcription responses and microRNA-directed post transcriptional mechanisms [130].

1,25-dihydroxyvitamins D and analogs have been reported to inhibit the proliferation of and induce the differentiation of a wide variety of cancer cell types, including human malignant melanoma [131]. This mechanism is carried out through the VDRs, which work as tumor suppressors. Laboratory experiments show that in keratinocytes lacking VDR, there is an increased expression of oncogenes and decreased expression of tumor suppressors, which predisposes the VDR deficient mice to skin cancer formation [132]. Vitamin D3 and its analogs also demonstrate moderate antiangiogenic properties, similar to those of all-trans retinoic acid [133].

Therefore, vitamin D signaling can protect the skin from cancer formation by controlling keratinocyte proliferation and differentiation by suppressing activation of the Hedgehog signaling pathway (Hh pathway) following UVR exposure [133], facilitating DNA repair, and preventing neo-vascularization [134–136].

Analogs of vitamin D belong to the class of potent inducers of differentiation of human cancer cell lines [137]. Vitamin D and its analogs induce apoptosis when combined with retinoid acid [138] through the reduction of bcl-2 protein, a pro-apoptotic protein, and increase in p53 and p21WAF-1, both tumor suppressors [139]. Because of this synergism and known chemopreventive activity of retinoids, the combination of vitamin D analogs and retinoids could be indicated for chemoprevention of carcinomas in high risk groups (xeroderma pigmentosum, arsenical keratoses, early actinic keratoses developing in chronic radiodermitis or in patients with epidermolysis bullosa dystrophica). Lastly, when combined with various cytokines, Vitamin D has an antitumor effect [140], and may be an effective chemoprevention strategy. Despite success in animal experiments, studies with Squamous-cell carcinoma (SCC) failed to respond to 1.25(OH)$_2$D$_3$, a Vitamin D analog, and showed no change in VDR gene expression compared to normal keratinocytes [133]. To ameliorate this issue, perhaps some modifications of the compounds or new derivatives of vitamin D may prove more efficacious and should be introduced in clinical practice [141].

Polyphenols

Research is human cell cultures indicates extensive anticancer properties of resveratrol, a natural phenol found in red grapes, red wine, peanuts, and pines [142]. Through anti-angiogenic, pro-apoptotic, and antioxidant behavior in skin cancers, resveratrol has proved to be a successful chemopreventive agent in murine models [143–145]. Its anti-angiogenic activity is linked to the down regulation of vascular endothelial growth factor (VEGF), a critical protein in the recruitment of new blood vessels, and the up-regulation of the p53 tumor suppressor [142, 143].

Studies on human melanoma show that resveratrol also decreases expression of thrombospondin 1 (TSP1), hypoxia inducible factor-1α (HIF-1α), and toll-like receptor 4 (TLR4), proteins heavily implicated in angiogenesis [143, 146, 147]. The pro-apoptotic effects of resveratrol are linked to a down regulation of Bcl-2, an anti-apoptotic protein and NF-kB, a pro-inflammatory transcription factor [148]. The inhibition of lipoxygenase and cyclooxygenase are responsible for the antioxidant behavior of resveratrol [144], further enhancing its anticancer activity. Despite the aforementioned positive characteristics, in some situations, resveratrol has also exhibited pro-angiogenic properties such as in peri-infarct myocardium tissues [149]. Numerous studies on both animal and human cell line models have been successful in confirming the chemopreventive potential of resveratrol. However, small scale clinical trials have failed to improve the bioavailability and identify the exact mechanisms of actions of resveratrol [145]. Thus, further investigation into resveratrol and its chemopreventive properties is warranted to further understand its effects and improve its efficacy in human cancer.

Myricetin is another dietary polyphenol flavonoid that exhibits anticancer properties. Commonly found in vegetables, fruits, nuts, berries, tea, and red wine [150–152], myricetin demonstrates antioxidant and anti-angiogenic properties [153]. Similar to resveratrol, some studies show that it inhibits VEGF by directly decreasing expression of associated regulatory proteins HIF-1α, p-Akt, and ribosomal protein S6 Kinase (p70S6K) [154, 155]. Other studies point the anti-angiogenic effects of myricetin to its increased transcription of p21, a cell cycle regulatory gene that can therefore down regulate HIF-1α and VEGF expression [146, 156]. Its antioxidant behavior is related to its inhibition of COX-2 expression by targeting the NF-kB inflammatory pathway [157].

among many others including MAPK [158], Akt [159], Fyn [160], and JAK/STAT3 [161] oncogenic pathways. This widespread effect on multiple signaling pathways shows the potential of myricetin as a chemopreventive agent, and should be further investigated in human clinical trials.

A compound in the polyphenol class which has shown promise is a very low molecular weight polyphenol, Honokiol. Honokiol is the active principle of Magnolia extract [162] and is orally bioavailable compared to curcumin. It has previously demonstrated both antiangiogenic and antitumor activity in a number of preclinical studies [163]. In a study by Battle et al, honokiol was shown to cause apoptosis preferentially in cells derived from chronic lymphocytic leukemia patients sparing the normal lymphocytic cells. They noted an upregulation of Bax protein with no effect on anti-apoptotic protein bcl2 [164]. Honokiol has shown to decreases activation of NF-κB and Akt signaling mechanisms and thus a decreases in levels of NF-κB target genes like VEGF, matrix metalloproteinase-9, ICAM-1, COX-2 [165]. More recently, it has been shown to have chemopreventive activity in UV induced skin cancer. Among the established mechanisms of action of honokiol is induction of the mitochondrial enzyme sirt 3. This can act as an antioxidant in normal cells by induced mitochondrial fusion, while it can induce reactive oxygen in premalignant and malignant cells with defective mitochondria, thus potentially leading to selective death of cells with mitochondrial defects [166].

Summary

Skin cancer continues to affect an increasing number of people in the United States. Even though there is a number of commercially available natural and synthetic substance and an equally large numbers under study for chemopreventive mechanisms, the results leaves much to be desired. Further research is required to substantiate the chemopreventive effects of substances discussed in this chapter. A major obstacle to the use of chemopreventive natural products is the formulation of these compounds in a stable form that can be topically delivered to the basal layer of the epidermis and upper dermis to inhibit angiogenesis and carcinogenesis.

References

1. Robinson JK. Sun exposure, sun protection, and vitamin D. JAMA. 2005;294(12):1541.
2. Siegel RL, Miller KD, Jemal A. Cancer statistics, 2016. CA Cancer J Clin. 2016;66(1):7–30.
3. Rees JR, Scot Zens M, Gui J, Celaya MO, Riddle BL, Karagas MR. Non melanoma skin cancer and subsequent cancer risk. PLoS One. 2014;9(6):e99674.
4. American Cancer Society. Cancer facts & figures 2016. Atlanta: American Cancer Society; 2016.
5. Jemal A, Siegel R, Ward E, Hao Y, Xu J, Thun MJ. Cancer statistics, 2009. CA Cancer J Clin. 2009;59(4):225–49.
6. What you need to know about melanoma and other skin cancers. National Cancer Institute. http://www.cancer.gov/publications/patient-education/wyntk-skin-cancer. Accessed 2 Apr 2016.
7. Smith JG, Davidson EA, Sams WM, Clark RD. Alterations in human dermal connective tissue with age and chronic sun damage. J Invest Dermatol. 1962;39(4):347–50.
8. Chung JH, Seo JY, Choi HR, Lee MK, Youn CS, Rhie G-E, et al. Modulation of skin collagen metabolism in aged and photoaged human skin in vivo. J Invest Dermatol. 2001;117(5):1218–24.
9. Kvaskoff M, Weinstein P. Are some melanomas caused by artificial light? Med Hypotheses. 2010;75(3):305–11.
10. Troll W, Wiesner R. The role of oxygen radicals as a possible mechanism of tumor promotion. Annu Rev Pharmacol Toxicol. 1985;25(1):509–28.
11. Gruijl FRD. Photocarcinogenesis: UVA vs UVB. Methods Enzymol. 2000;319:359–66.
12. Bachelor MA, Bowden G. UVA-mediated activation of signaling pathways involved in skin tumor promotion and progression. Semin Cancer Biol. 2004;14(2):131–8.
13. Cheng KC, Cahill DS, Kasai H, Nishimura S, Loeb LA. 8-Hydroxyguanine, an abundant form of oxidative DNA damage, causes G→T and A→C substitutions. J Biol Chem. 1992;267:166–72.
14. Nandakumar V, Vaid M, Tollefsbol TO, Katiyar SK. Aberrant DNA hypermethylation patterns lead to transcriptional silencing of tumor suppressor genes in UVB-exposed skin and UVB-induced skin tumors of mice. Carcinogenesis. 2011;32(4):597–604.
15. Tong X, Mirzoeva S, Veliceasa D, Bridgeman BB, Fitchev P, Cornwell ML, et al. Chemopreventive apigenin controls UVB-induced cutaneous proliferation and angiogenesis through HuR and thrombospondin-1. Oncotarget. 2014;5(22):11413–27.
16. Kang NJ, Jung SK, Lee KW, Lee HJ. Myricetin is a potent chemopreventive phytochemical in skin carcinogenesis. Ann N Y Acad Sci. 2011;1229(1):124–32.
17. Einspahr JG, Thomas TL, Saboda K, Nickolof BJ, Warneke J, Curiel-Lewandrowski C, et al. Expression of vascular endothelial growth factor in early cutaneous melanocytic lesion progression. Cancer. 2007;110(11):2519–27.
18. Wogan GN, Hecht SS, Felton JS, Conney AH, Loeb LA. Environmental and chemical carcinogenesis. Semin Cancer Biol. 2004;14(6):473–86.
19. Einspahr JG, Stratton SP, Bowden G, Alberts DS. Chemoprevention of human skin cancer. Crit Rev Oncol Hematol. 2002;41(3):269–85.
20. Adami J, Gabel H, Lindelof B, Ekström K, Rydh B, Glimelius B, et al. Cancer risk following organ transplantation: A nationwide cohort study in Sweden. Br J Cancer. 2003;89:1221.

21. Gruber SA, Gillingham K, Sothern RB, Stephanian E, Matas AJ, Dunn DL. De novo cancer in cyclosporine-treated and non-cyclosporine-treated adult primary renal allograft recipients. Clin Transplant. 1994;8:388.
22. Petronzelli F, Sollima D, Coppola G, Martini-Neri ME, Neri G, Genuardi M. CDKN2A germline splicing mutation affecting both p16(ink4) and p14(arf) RNA processing in a melanoma/neurofibroma kindred. Genes Chromosomes Cancer. 2001;31(4):398–401.
23. Sporn MB. Carcinogenesis and cancer: Different perspectives on the same disease. Cancer Res. 1991;51:6215–8.
24. Marks F, Fürstenberger G. Cancer chemoprevention through interruption of multistage carcinogenesis. Eur J Cancer. 2000;36(3):314–29.
25. Flora SD, Ferguson LR. Overview of mechanisms of cancer chemopreventive agents. Mutat Res/Fundam Mol Mech Mutagen. 2005;591(1-2):8–15.
26. Bonovas S, Tsantes A, Drosos T, Sitaras NM. Cancer chemoprevention: A summary of the current evidence. Anticancer Res. 2008;28(3B):1857–66.
27. Lippman SM, Lee JJ, Sabichi AL. Cancer Chemoprevention: Progress and Promise. JNCI J Nati Cancer Inst. 1998;90(20):1514–28.
28. Rao C, Reddy BS. NSAIDs and Chemoprevention. Curr Cancer Drug Targets CCDT. 2004;4(1):29–42.
29. Hudlicka O. Growth of capillaries in skeletal and cardiac muscle. Circ Res. 1982;50(4):451–61.
30. Nagy JA, Chang S-H, Dvorak AM, Dvorak HF. Why are tumour blood vessels abnormal and why is it important to know? Br J Cancer. 2009;100(6):865–9.
31. Folkman J. Tumor angiogenesis. Adv Cancer Res. 1985;175–203
32. Marks F, Müller-Decker K, Fürstenberger G. A causal relationship between unscheduled eicosanoid signaling and tumor development: Cancer chemoprevention by inhibitors of arachidonic acid metabolism. Toxicology. 2000;153(1–3):11–26.
33. Melder RJ, Koenig GC, Witwer BP, Safabakhsh N, Munn LL, Jain RK. During angiogenesis, vascular endothelial growth factor regulate natural killer cell adhesion to tumor endothelium. Nat Med. 1996;2(9):992–7.
34. Arbiser JL, Byers HR, Cohen C, Arbeit J. Altered basic fibroblast growth factor expression in common epidermal neoplasms: Examination with in situ hybridization and immunohistochemistry. J Am Acad Dermatol. 2000 Jun;42(6):973–7.
35. Logie A, Dunois-Larde C, Rosty C, Levrel O, Blanche M, Ribeiro A, et al. Activating mutations of the tyrosine kinase receptor FGFR3 are associated with benign skin tumors in mice and humans. Hum Mol Genet. 2005;14:1153–60.
36. Breier G, Albrecht U, Sterrer S, Risau W. Expression of vascular endothelial growth factor during embryonic angiogenesis and endothelial cell differentiation. Development. 1992;114:521–32.
37. Li WW, Casey R, Gonzalez EM, Folkman J. Angiostatic steroids potentiated by sulfated cyclodextrins inhibit corneal neovascularization. Invest Ophthalmol Vis Sci. 1991;32(11):2898–905.
38. Miller JW, Adamis AP, Shima DT, D'amore PA, Moulton RS, O'reilly MS, et al. Vascular endothelial growth factor/vascular permeability factor is temporally and spatially correlated with ocular angiogenesis in a primate model. Retina. 1995;15(2):174.
39. Takahashi K, Mulliken JB, Kozakewich HP, Rogers RA, Folkman J, Ezekowitz RA. Cellular markers that distinguish the phases of hemangioma during infancy and childhood. J Clin Invest. 1994;93(6):2357–64.
40. Peacock DJ. Angiogenesis inhibition suppresses collagen arthritis. J Exp Med. 1992;175(4):1135–8.
41. Rothstein R. Safety profiles of leading nonsteroidal anti-inflammatory drugs. Am J Med. 1998;105(5):39S–43S.
42. Mcdonald JJ. A single amino acid difference between cyclooxygenase-1 (COX-1) and -2(COX-2) reverses the selectivity of COX-2 specific inhibitors. J Biol Chem. 1996;271(26):15810–4.

43. Williams CS, DuBois RN. Prostaglandin endoperoxide synthase: Why two isoforms? Am J Physiol. 1996;270(3 Pt 1):G393–400.
44. Surh YJ, Chun KS. Cancer chemopreventive effects of curcumin. Adv Exp Med Biol. 2007;595:149–72.
45. Liu CH, Chang SH, Narko K, Trifan OC, Wu MT, Smith E, et al. Overexpression of cyclooxygenase-2 is sufficient to induce tumorigenesis in transgenic mice. J Biol Chem. 2001;276(21):18563–9.
46. Martin SP, Ulrich CD. Pancreatic cancer surveillance in a high-risk cohort. Is it worth the cost? Med Clin North Am. 2000;84:739. xii.
47. Vainio H, Morgan G. Ann Chir Gynaecol. 2000;89:173.
48. Harris RE. Cyclooxygenase-2 (cox-2) blockade in the chemoprevention of cancers of the colon, breast, prostate, and lung. Inflammopharmacology. 2009;17(2):55–67.
49. Kelley D. Benzo[a] pyrene up-regulates cyclooxygenase-2 gene expression in oral epithelial cells. Carcinogenesis. 1997;18(4):795–9.
50. Song S, Lippman SM, Zou Y, Ye X, Ajani JA, Xu X-C. Induction of cyclooxygenase-2 by benzo[a]pyrene diol epoxide through inhibition of retinoic acid receptor-β2 expression. Oncogene. 2005;24(56):8268–76.
51. Karmali RA. Dietary fatty acids, COX-2 blockade, and carcinogenesis. In: Harris RE, ed. COX-2 blockade in cancer prevention and therapy. Totowa, NJ: Humana Press; 2002. pp. 3–12.
52. Burd R, Choy H, Dicker A. Potential for inhibitors of cyclooxygenase-2 to enhance tumor radioresponse. In: Harris RE, ed. COX-2 blockade in cancer prevention and therapy. Totowa, NJ: Humana Press; 2002. pp. 301–311.
53. Buckman S. COX-2 expression is induced by UVB exposure in human skin: Implications for the development of skin cancer. Carcinogenesis. 1998;19(5):723–9.
54. Jaimes EA, Tian R-X, Pearse D, Raij L. Up-regulation of glomerular COX-2 by angiotensin II: Role of reactive oxygen species. Kidney Int. 2005;68(5):2143–53.
55. Chang Y-WE, Putzer K, Ren L, Kaboord B, Chance TW, Qoronfleh MW, et al. Differential regulation of cyclooxygenase 2 expression by small GTPases Ras, Rac1, and RhoA. J Cell Biochem. 2005;96(2):314–29.
56. Coffey RJ, Hawkey CJ, Damstrup L, Graves-Deal R, Daniel VC, Dempsey PJ, et al. Epidermal growth factor receptor activation induces nuclear targeting of cyclooxygenase-2, basolateral release of prostaglandins, and mitogenesis in polarizing colon cancer cells. Proc Natl Acad Sci. 1997;94(2):657–62.
57. Chang YJ, Wu MS, Lin JT, Chen CC. Helicobacter pylori-induced invasion and angiogenesis of gastric cells is mediated by cyclooxygenase-2 induction through TLR2/TLR9 and promoter regulation. J Immunol. 2005;175(12):8242–52.
58. Singh A, Sharma H, Salhan S, Gupta SD, Bhatla N, Jain S, et al. Evaluation of expression of apoptosis-related proteins and their correlation with HPV, telomerase activity, and apoptotic index in cervical cancer. Pathobiology. 2004;71(6):314–22.
59. Cheng AS-L, Chan HL-Y, Leung WK, To KF, Go MY-Y, Chan JY-H, et al. Expression of HBx and COX-2 in chronic hepatitis B, cirrhosis and hepatocellular carcinoma: Implication of HBx in upregulation of COX-2. Mod Pathol. 2004;17(10):1169–79.
60. Kaul R, Verma SC, Murakami M, Lan K, Choudhuri T, Robertson ES. Epstein-Barr virus protein can upregulate cyclo-oxygenase-2 expression through association with the suppressor of metastasis Nm23-H1. J Virol. 2006;80(3):1321–31.
61. Harris RE, Beebe-Donk J, Alshafie GA. Reduction in the risk of human breast cancer by selective cyclooxygenase-2 (COX-2) inhibitors. BMC Cancer. 2006;6(1):27.
62. Zhuang Z-H, Tsao S-W, Deng W, Wang J-D, Xia HH-X, He H, et al. Early upregulation of cyclooxygenase-2 in human papillomavirus type 16 and telomerase-induced immortalization of human esophageal epithelial cells. J Gastroenterol Hepatol. 2008;23(10):1613–20.
63. Gurpinar E, Grizzle WE, Piazza GA. NSAIDs inhibit tumorigenesis, but how? Clin Cancer Res. 2013;20(5):1104–13.

64. Harris RE, Kasbari S, Farrar WB. Prospective study of nonsteroidal anti-inflammatory drugs and breast cancer. Oncol Rep. 1999;6(1):71–3.
65. Vane JR. Inhibition of prostaglandin synthesis as a mechanism of action for aspirin-like drugs. Nat New Biol. 1971;231(25):232–5.
66. Bentham Science Publisher, Sarkar FH, Adsule S, Li Y, Padhye S. Back to the Future: COX-2 Inhibitors for Chemoprevention and Cancer Therapy. MRMC Mini-Rev Med Chem. 2007;7(6):599–608.
67. Berg J, Christoph T, Widerna M, Bodenteich A. Isoenzyme-specific cyclooxygenase inhibitors: A whole cell assay system using the human erythroleukemic cell line HEL and the human monocytic cell line Mono Mac 6. J Pharmacol Toxicol Methods. 1997;37(4):179–86.
68. Elwich-Flis S, Soltysiak-Pawluczuk D, Splawinski J. Anti-angiogenic and apoptotic effects of metabolites of sulindac on chick embryo chorioallantoic membrane. Hybrid Hybridomics. 2003;22:55–60.
69. Skopinska-Rozewska E, Piazza GA, Sommer E, Pamukcu R, Barcz E, Filewska M, et al. Inhibition of angiogenesis by sulindac and its sulfone metabolite (FGN-1): A potential mechanism for their antineoplastic properties. Int J Tissue React. 1998;20:85–9.
70. Lin HP, Kulp SK, Tseng PH, Yang YT, Yang CC, Chen CS, et al. Growth inhibitory effects of celecoxib in human umbilical vein endothelial cells are mediated through G1 arrest via multiple signaling mechanisms. Mol Cancer Ther. 2004;3:1671–80.
71. Wei D, Wang L, He Y, Xiong HQ, Abbruzzese JL, Xie K. Celecoxib inhibits vascular endothelial growth factor expression in and reduces angiogenesis and metastasis of human pancreatic cancer via suppression of Sp1 transcription factor activity. Cancer Res. 2004;64:2030–8.
72. Lee HC, Park IC, Park MJ, An S, Woo SH, Jin HO, et al. Sulindac and its metabolites inhibit invasion of glioblastoma cells via down-regulation of Akt/PKB and MMP-2. J Cell Biochem. 2005;94:597–610.
73. Keller JJ, Offerhaus GJ, Polak M, Goodman SN, Zahurak ML, Hylind LM, et al. Rectal epithelial apoptosis in familial adenomatous polyposis patients treated with sulindac. Gut. 1999;45:822–8.
74. Kolligs FT, Bommer G, Goke B. Wnt/beta-catenin/tcf signaling: A critical pathway in gastrointestinal tumorigenesis. Digestion. 2002;66:131–44.
75. Tinsley HN, Gary BD, Keeton AB, Lu W, Li Y, Piazza GA. Inhibition of PDE5 by sulindac sulfide selectively induces apoptosis and attenuates oncogenic Wnt/betacatenin- mediated transcription in human breast tumor cells. Cancer Prev Res (Phila). 2011;4:1275–84.
76. Yin MJ, Yamamoto Y, Gaynor RB. The anti-inflammatory agents aspirin and salicylate inhibit the activity of I(kappa)B kinase-beta. Nature. 1998;396:77–80.
77. Yamamoto Y, Yin MJ, Lin KM, Gaynor RB. Sulindac inhibits activation of the NF-kappaB pathway. J Biol Chem. 1999;274:27307–14.
78. Fosslien E. Biochemistry of cyclooxygenase (COX)-2 inhibitors and molecular pathology of COX-2 in neoplasia. Crit Rev Clin Lab Sci. 2000;37(5):431–502.
79. Marnett LJ. The COXIB experience: A look in the rearview mirror. Annu Rev Pharmacol Toxicol. 2009;49:265–90.
80. Gottlieb S. COX 2 inhibitors may increase risk of heart attack. BMJ. 2001;323:471.
81. Bree AF. Shah MR; BCNS Colloquium Group. Consensus statement from the first international colloquium on basal cell nevus syndrome (BCNS). Am J Med Genet A. 2011;155A(9):2091–7.
82. Reifenberger J, Wolter M, Knobbe CB, Köhler B, Schönicke A, Scharwächter C, et al. Somatic mutations in the PTCH, SMOH, SUFUH and TP53 genes in sporadic basal cell carcinoma. Br J Dermatol. 2005;152:43–51.
83. Fecher LA, Sharfman WH. Advanced basal cell carcinoma, the hedgehog pathway, and treatment options - role of smoothened inhibitors. Biologics. 2015;9:129–40.
84. Piérard-Franchimont C, Hermanns-Lê T, Paquet P, Herfs M, Delvenne P, Piérard GE. Hedgehog- and mTOR-targeted therapies for advanced basal cell carcinomas. Future Oncol. 2015;11(22):2997–3002.

85. Thangapazham RL, Sharma A, Maheshwari RK. Beneficial role of curcumin in skin diseases. Adv Exp Med Biol. 2007;595:343–57.
86. Sa G, Das T. Anti cancer effects of curcumin: Cycle of life and death. Cell Div. 2008;3(1):14.
87. Azuine MA, Bhide SV. Chemopreventive effect of turmeric against stomach and skin tumors induced by chemical carcinogens in Swiss mice. Nutr Cancer. 1992;17(1):77–83.
88. Singh M, Suman S, Shukla Y. New enlightenment of skin cancer chemoprevention through Phytochemicals: In vitro and in vivo studies and the underlying mechanisms. Biomed Res Int. 2014:243452.
89. Dinarello CA. The paradox of pro-inflammatory cytokines in cancer. Cancer Metastasis Rev. 2006;25(3):307–13.
90. Kunnumakkara AB, Anand P, Aggarwal BB. Curcumin inhibits proliferation, invasion, angiogenesis and metastasis of different cancers through interaction with multiple cell signaling proteins. Cancer Lett. 2008;269(2):199–225.
91. Chun K-S. Curcumin inhibits phorbol ester-induced expression of cyclooxygenase-2 in mouse skin through suppression of extracellular signal-regulated kinase activity and NF- B activation. Carcinogenesis. 2003;24(9):1515–24.
92. Bhandarkar SS, Arbiser JL. Curcumin as an inhibitor of angiogenesis. Adv Exp Med Biol. 2007;595:185–95.
93. Grandjean-Laquerriere A, Gangloff SC, Naour RL, Trentesaux C, Hornebeck W, Guenounou M. relative contribution of NF-Kb and AP-1 in the modulation by curcumin and pyrrolidine dithiocarbamate of the UVB-induced cytokine expression by keratinocytes. Cytokine. 2002;18(3):168–77.
94. Kunnumakkara AB, Guha S, Krishnan S, Diagaradjane P, Gelovani J, Aggarwal BB. Curcumin potentiates antitumor activity of gemcitabine in an orthotopic model of pancreatic cancer through suppression of proliferation, angiogenesis, and inhibition of nuclear factor-B-regulated gene products. Cancer Res. 2007;67(8):3853–61.
95. Lin YG, Kunnumakkara AB, Nair A, Merritt WM, Han LY, Armaiz-Pena GN, et al. Curcumin inhibits tumor growth and angiogenesis in ovarian carcinoma by targeting the nuclear factor-B pathway. Clin Cancer Res. 2007;13(11):3423–30.
96. Arbiser JL, Klauber N, Rohan R, van Leeuwen R, Huang MT, Fisher C. Curcumin is an in vivo inhibitor of angiogenesis. Mol Med. 1998;4(6):376–83.
97. Cho J-W, Park K, Kweon GR, Jang B-C, Baek W-K, Suh M-H, et al. Curcumin inhibits the expression of COX-2 in UVB-irradiated human keratinocytes (HaCaT) by inhibiting activation of AP-1: p38 MAP kinase and JNK as potential upstream targets. Exp Mol Med. 2005;37(3):186–92.
98. Shoba G, Joy D, Joseph T, Majeed M, Rajendran R, Srinivas P. Influence of piperine on the pharmacokinetics of curcumin in animals and human volunteers. Planta Med. 1998;64(04):353–6.
99. Gu Z, Shan K, Chen H, Chen YQ. n-3 Polyunsaturated fatty acids and their role in cancer chemoprevention. Curr Pharmacol Rep. 2015;1:283–94.
100. Wang W, Zhu J, Lyu F, Panigrahy D, Ferrara KW, Hammock B, et al. ω-3 Polyunsaturated fatty acids-derived lipid metabolites on angiogenesis, inflammation and cancer. Prostaglandins Other Lipid Mediat. 2014;113-115:13–20.
101. Serini S, Fasano E, Celleno L, Cittadini A, Calviello G. Potential of long-chain n-3 polyunsaturated fatty acids in melanoma prevention. Nutr Rev. 2014;72(4):255–66.
102. Black H, Rhodes L. Potential benefits of omega-3 fatty acids in non-melanoma skin cancer. J Clin Med JCM. 2016;5(2):23.
103. Pardini RS. Nutritional intervention with omega-3 fatty acids enhances tumor response to anti-neoplastic agents. Chem Biol Interact. 2006;162(2):89–105.
104. Serini S, Donato V, Piccioni E, Trombino S, Monego G, Toesca A, et al. Docosahexaenoic acid reverts resistance to UV-induced apoptosis in human keratinocytes: Involvement of COX-2 and HuR. J Nutr Biochem. 2011;22(9):874–85.
105. Serini S, Fasano E, Piccioni E, Monego G, Cittadini ARM, Celleno L, et al. DHA induces apoptosis and differentiation in human melanoma cells in vitro: Involvement of

HuR-mediated COX-2 mRNA stabilization and β-catenin nuclear translocation. Carcinogenesis. 2011;33(1):164–73.

106. Albino AP et al. Cell cycle arrest and apoptosis of melanoma cells by docosahexaenoic acid: Association with decreased pRb phosphorylation. Cancer Res. 2000;60:4139–45.

107. Reich R, Royce L, Martin GR. Eicosapentaenoic acid reduces the invasive and metastatic activities of malignant tumor cells. Biochem Biophys Res Commun. 1989;160:559–64.

108. Serini S, Fasano E, Piccioni E, Cittadini ARM, Calviello G. Dietary n-3 polyunsaturated fatty acids and the paradox of their health benefits and potential harmful effects. Chem Res Toxicol. 2011;24:2093–105.

109. Pilkington SM et al. Randomized controlled trial of oral omega-3 PUFA in solar-simulated radiation-induced suppression of human cutaneous immune responses. Am J Clin Nutr. 2013;97:646–52.

110. Li K, Huang T, Zheng J, Wu K, Li D. Effect of marine-derived n-3 polyunsaturated fatty acids on C-reactive protein, interleukin 6 and tumor necrosis factor α: a meta-analysis. PLoS One. 2014;9(2):1–28.

111. Vara-Messler M et al. A potential role of PUFAs and COXIBs in cancer chemoprevention. Prostaglandins Other Lipid Mediat. 2015;120:97–102.

112. Wen B et al. n-3 Polyunsaturated fatty acids decrease mucosal/epidermal reactions and enhance antitumour effect of ionising radiation with inhibition of tumour angiogenesis. Br J Cancer. 2003;89:1102–7.

113. Siddiqui RA, Harvey KA, Zaloga GP, Stillwell W. Modulation of lipid rafts by Omega-3 fatty acids in inflammation and cancer: Implications for use of lipids during nutrition support. Nutr Clin Pract. 2007;22:74–88.

114. Im D-S. Omega-3 fatty acids in anti-inflammation (pro-resolution) and GPCRs. Prog Lipid Res. 2012;51:232–7.

115. Fennema O. Fennema's food chemistry. Boca Raton: CRC Press Taylor & Francis; 2008. p. 454–5.

116. Lobo GP, Hessel S, Eichinger A, et al. ISX is a retinoic acid-sensitive gatekeeper that controls intestinal beta,beta-carotene absorption and vitamin A production. FASEB J. 2010;24(6): 1656–66.

117. Narisawa T, Reddy BS, Wong CQ, Weisburger JH. Effect of vitamin A deficiency on rat colon carcinogenesis by N-methyl -N'-nitro-N-nitrosogua- nidine. Cancer Res. 1976;36(4):1379–83.

118. Fuchs E, Green H. Regulation of terminal differentiation of cultured human keratinocytes by vitamin A. Cell. 1981;25(3):617–25.

119. Weinstock MA, Bingham SF, Digiovanna JJ, et al. Tretinoin and the prevention of keratinocyte carcinoma (Basal and squamous cell carcinoma of the skin): A Veterans Affairs randomized chemoprevention trial. J Invest Dermatol. 2012;132(6):1583–90.

120. Zhang C, Duvic M. Retinoids: Therapeutic applications and mechanisms of action in cutaneous T-cell lymphoma. Dermatol Ther. 2003;16(4):322–30.

121. Aggarwal S, Kim SW, Cheon K, Tabassam FH, Yoon JH, Koo JS. Nonclassical action of retinoic acid on the activation of the cAMP response element- binding protein in normal human bronchial epithelial cells. Mol Biol Cell. 2006;17(2):566–75.

122. Faria TN, Mendelsohn C, Chambon P, Gudas LJ. The targeted disruption of both alleles of RARbeta(2) in F9 cells results in the loss of retinoic acid- associated growth arrest. J Biol Chem. 1999;274(38):26783–8.

123. Costa A, Formelli F, Chiesa F, Decensi A, De Palo G, Veronesi U. Prospects of chemoprevention of human cancers with the synthetic retinoid fenretinide. Cancer Res. 1994;54(7 Suppl):2032s–37ss.

124. Han J, Jiao L, Lu Y, Sun Z, Gu QM, Scanlon KJ. Evaluation of N-4-(hydrox- ycarbophenyl) retinamide as a cancer prevention agent and as a cancer chemotherapeutic agent. In Vivo. 1990;4(3):153–60.

125. Subbaramaiah K, Morris PG, Zhou XK, Morrow M, Du B, Giri D, et al. Increased Levels of COX-2 and prostaglandin E2 contribute to elevated aromatase expression in inflamed breast tissue of obese women. Cancer Discov. 2012;2(4):356–65.

126. Papi A, Carolis SD, Bertoni S, Storci G, Sceberras V, Santini D, et al. PPARγ and RXR ligands disrupt the inflammatory cross-talk in the hypoxic breast cancer stem cells niche. J Cell Physiol. 2014;229(11):1595–606.

127. Lotan R. Retinoids in cancer chemoprevention. FASEB J. 1996;10:1031–9.

128. Bouillon R, Okamura WH, Norman AW. Structure-function relationships m the vitamin D endocrine system. Endocr Rev. 1995;16:200–57.

129. Dietary reference intakes for thiamin, riboflavin, niacin, vitamin B 6, folate, vitamin B 12, pantothenic acid, biotin, and choline: A report of the standing committee on the scientific evaluation of dietary reference intakes and its panel on folate, other B vitamins, and choline and subcommittee on upper reference levels of nutrients. Q Rev Biol. 2003;78(3):384–5. http://www.journals.uchicago.edu/doi/abs/10.1086/380067; https://www.ncbi.nlm.nih.gov/books/NBK114310/.

130. Moore DD et al. International Union of Pharmacology. LXII. The NR1H and NR1I receptors: Constitutive androstane receptor, pregnene X receptor, farnesoid X receptor alpha, farnesoid X receptor beta, liver X receptor alpha, liver X receptor beta, and vitamin D receptor. Pharmacol Rev. 2006;58:742–59.

131. Skowronski RJ, Peehl DM, Feldman D. Vitamin D and prostate cancer: 1,25 dihydroxyvitamin D3 receptors and actions in human prostate cancer cell lines. Endocrinology. 1993;132:1952–60.

132. Jiang YJ, Bikle DD. LncRNA profiling reveals new mechanism for VDR protection against skin cancer formation. J Steroid Biochem Mol Biol. 2014;144:87–90.

133. Majewski S, Skopinska M, Marczak M, Szmurlo A, Bollag W, Jablonska S. Vitamin D3 is potent inhibitor of tumor cell-induced angiogenesis. Investig Dermatol Symp Proc. 1996;1(1):97–101.

134. Oikawa T, Hirotani K, Ogasawara H, Katayama T, Nakamura O, Iwaguchi T. Inhibition of angiogenesis by vitamin D3 analogues. Eur J Pharmacol. 1990;178(2):247–50.

135. Majewski S, Szmurlo A, Marczak M, Jablonska S, Bollag W. Inhibition of tumor cell-induced angiogenesis by retinoids, 1,25-dihydroxyvitamin D3 and their combination. Cancer Lett. 1993;75:35–9.

136. Majewski S, Marczak M, Szmurlo A, Jablonska S, Bollag W. Retinoids, Interferon α, 1,25-dihydroxyvitamin D3 and their combination inhibit angiogenesis induced by non-HPV-harboring tumor cell lines. RARα mediates the antiangiogenic effect of retinoids. Cancer Lett. 1995;89:117–24.

137. Binderup L, Latini S, Binderup E, Bretting C, Calverley M, Hansen K. 20-EPI-vitamin D3 analogues: A novel class of potent regulators of cell growth and immune responses. Biochem Pharmacol. 1991;42(8):1569–75.

138. James SY, Williams MA, Newland AC, Colston KW. Leukemia cell differentiation: Cellular and molecular interactions of retinoids and vitamin D. Gen Pharmacol. 1999;32:143–54.

139. James SY, Mackay AG, Colston KW. Effects of 1,25 dihydroxyvitamin D3 and its analogues on induction of apoptosis in breast cancer cells. J Steroid Biochem Mol Biol. 1996;58:395–401.

140. Majewski S, Marczak M, Szmurlo A, Jablonska S, Bollag W. Interleukin-12 inhibits angiogenesis induced by human tumor cell lines in vivo. J Invest Dermatol. 1996;106:1114–8.

141. Majewski S, Kutner A, Jabłonska S. Vitamin D analogs in cutaneous malignancies. Curr Pharm Des. 2000;6:829–38.

142. Miller NJ, Rice-Evans CA. Antioxidant activity of resveratrol in red wine. Clin Chem. 1998;41:1789.

143. Lin M-T. Inhibition of vascular endothelial growth factor-induced angiogenesis by resveratrol through interruption of Src-dependent vascular endothelial cadherin tyrosine phosphorylation. Mol Pharmacol. 2003;64(5):1029–36.

144. Niles RM, Mcfarland M, Weimer MB, Redkar A, Fu Y-M, Meadows GG. Resveratrol is a potent inducer of apoptosis in human melanoma cells. Cancer Lett. 2003;190(2):157–63.
145. Athar M, Back JH, Tang X, Kim KH, Kopelovich L, Bickers DR, Kim AL. Resveratrol: A review of preclinical studies for human cancer prevention. Toxicol Appl Pharmacol. 2007;224:274–83.
146. Wu H, Liang X, Fang Y, Qin X, Zhang Y, Liu J. Resveratrol inhibits hypoxia-induced metastasis potential enhancement by restricting hypoxia-induced factor-1α expression in colon carcinoma cells. Biomed Pharmacother. 2008;62(9):613–21.
147. Yusuf N, Nasti TH, Meleth S, Elmets CA. Resveratrol enhances cell-mediated immune response to DMBA through TLR4 and prevents DMBA induced cutaneous carcinogenesis. Mol Carcinog. 2009;48(8):713–23.
148. Pozo-Guisado E, Merino JM, Mulero-Navarro S, Lorenzo-Benayas MJ, Centeno F, Alvarez-Barrientos A, Fernandez-Salguero PM. Resveratrol-induced apoptosis in MCF-7 human breast cancer cells involves a caspase-independent mechanism with downregulation of Bcl-2 and NF-kappaB. Int J Cancer. 2005;115:74–84.
149. Kaga S, Zhan L, Matsumoto M, Maulik N. Resveratrol enhances neovascularization in the infarcted rat myocardium through the induction of thioredoxin-1, heme oxygenase-1 and vascular endothelial growth factor. J Mol Cell Cardiol. 2005;39(5):813–22.
150. Harnly JM, Doherty RF, Beecher GR, Holden JM, Haytowitz DB, Bhagwat S, et al. Flavonoid content of U.S. fruits, vegetables, and nuts. J Agric Food Chem. 2006;54(26):9966–77.
151. Ledda S, Sanna G, Manca G, Franco MA, Porcu A. Variability in flavonol content of grapes cultivated in two Mediterranean islands (Sardinia and Corsica). J Food Compos Anal. 2010;23(6):580–5.
152. Wang H, Helliwell K. Determination of flavonols in green and black tea leaves and green tea infusions by high-performance liquid chromatography. Food Res Int. 2001;34(2-3):223–7.
153. Ong KC, Khoo H-E. Biological effects of myricetin. Gen Pharmacol: Vasc Sys. 1997;29(2):121–6.
154. Huang H, Chen AY, Rojanasakul Y, Ye X, Rankin GO, Chen YC. Dietary compounds galangin and myricetin suppress ovarian cancer cell angiogenesis. J Funct Foods. 2015;15:464–75.
155. Jung SK, Lee KW, Byun S, Lee EJ, Kim JE, Bode AM, et al. Myricetin inhibits UVB-induced angiogenesis by regulating PI-3 kinase in vivo. Carcinogenesis. 2009;31(5):911–7.
156. Ghahremani MF, Goossens S, Nittner D, Bisteau X, Bartunkova S, Zwolinska A, et al. p53 promotes VEGF expression and angiogenesis in the absence of an intact p21-Rb pathway. Cell Death Differ. 2013;20(7):888–97.
157. Lee KM, Kang NJ, Han JH, Lee KW, Lee HJ. Myricetin down-regulates phorbol ester-induced cyclooxygenase-2 expression in mouse epidermal cells by blocking activation of nuclear factor kappa B. J Agric Food Chem. 2007;55(23):9678–84.
158. Lee KW, Kang NJ, Rogozin EA, Kim H-G, Cho YY, Bode AM, et al. Myricetin is a novel natural inhibitor of neoplastic cell transformation and MEK1. Carcinogenesis. 2007;28(9):1918–27.
159. Kumamoto T, Fujii M, Hou DX. Akt is a direct target for myricetin to inhibit cell transformation. Mol Cell Biochem. 2009;332(1-2):33–41.
160. Jung SK, Lee KW, Byun S, Kang NJ, Lim SH, Heo Y-S, et al. Myricetin Suppresses UVB-Induced Skin Cancer by Targeting Fyn. Cancer Res. 2008;68(14):6021–9.
161. Kumamoto T, Fujii M, Hou D-X. Myricetin directly targets JAK1 to inhibit cell transformation. Cancer Lett. 2009;275(1):17–26.
162. Fried LE, Arbiser JL. Honokiol, a multifunctional antiangiogenic and antitumor agent. Antioxid Redox Signal. 2009;11(5):1139–48.

163. Bai X, Cerimele F, Ushio-Fukai M, Waqas M, Campbell PM, Govindarajan B. Honokiol, a small molecular weight natural product, inhibits angiogenesis in vitro and tumor growth in vivo. J Biol Chem. 2003;278:35501–7.
164. Battle TE, Arbiser J, Frank DA. Blood. 2005;106(2):690–7.
165. Ahn KS, Sethi G, Shishodia S, Sung B, Arbiser JL, Aggarwal BB. Honokiol potentiates apoptosis, suppresses osteoclastogenesis, and inhibits invasion through modulation of nuclear factor-kappaB activation pathway. Mol Cancer Res. 2006;4:621–33.
166. Mędra A, Witkowska M, Majchrzak A, Cebula-Obrzut B, Bonner MY. 3, Robak T. pro-apoptotic activity of new honokiol/triphenylmethane analogues in B-cell lymphoid malignancies. Molecules. 2016;21(8):995.

Angiogenesis and Pathogenesis of Port Wine Stain and Infantile Hemangiomas

Wangcun Jia, Carol Cheng, Wenbin Tan, Martin C. Mihm Jr, and J. Stuart Nelson

Introduction

The vascular system maintains human homeostasis by providing nutrients, oxygen and hormones to trillions of cells in the body and removing metabolic wastes. The vascular system is composed of a complex network of arteries, arterioles, capillaries, venules, veins, and lymphatic vessels. The vasculature forms during the embryonic development stages and consists of two distinct cell types: (1) endothelial cells which form the endothelium, the interior surface of blood vessels; and (2) perivascular supporting cells, such as smooth muscle cells which form the wall of blood vessels, and pericytes, a key component of the neurovascular unit.

A vascular anomaly results when a developmental error or dysregulated developmental processes of the vascular system occur. Vascular anomalies are characterized by an increase in the number of vessels and/or enlargement of vessels. Abnormalities can affect one type of blood vessel, such as capillaries, or multiple types of blood vessels, such as arterioles and venules. Vascular anomalies can be either congenital,

W. Jia • W. Tan
Beckman Laser Institute, Department of Surgery, University of California,
Irvine, CA 92617, USA

C. Cheng • M.C. Mihm Jr
Department of Dermatology, Brigham and Women's Hospital, Harvard Institute of Medicine,
55 Fruit Street, Boston, MA 02115, USA
e-mail: mmihm@partners.org

J. Stuart Nelson (✉)
Beckman Laser Institute, Department of Surgery, University of California,
Irvine, CA 92617, USA

Department of Biomedical Engineering, University of California,
1002 Health Sciences Rd, Irvine, CA 92617, USA
e-mail: jsnelson@uci.edu

© Springer-Verlag London Ltd. 2017
J.L. Arbiser (ed.), *Angiogenesis-Based Dermatology*,
DOI 10.1007/978-1-4471-7314-4_8

which exist at birth or occur within weeks to years after birth, or non-congenital, which are caused by environmental factors such as trauma.

According to a classification scheme proposed by Mulliken and Glowacki [1] and the 1996 revision by the International Society for the Study of Vascular Anomalies (ISSVA), vascular anomalies can be divided into two categories: vascular malformations and vascular tumors. Vascular malformations have a normal endothelial cell cycle but the blood vessels are larger and/or the vessel number densities are higher in the lesions as compared to normal skin [2–4]. Vascular malformations are categorized by the type of affected blood vessels and, thus, there are capillary, venous, arterial, lymphatic or combined malformations. In contrast, the distinctive features of vascular tumors are endothelial cell proliferation and rapid postnatal growth followed by involution [2–4] . Some of the notable types of vascular tumors are: (a) hemangioma, (b) Kaposiform hemangioendothelioma, (c) tufted angioma, (d) pyogenic granuloma; and (e) hemangiopericytoma.

In this chapter, both types of vascular anomalies, port wine stain (PWS, vascular malformation) and infantile hemangiomas (IH, vascular tumor), will be discussed. Discussions will focus on the pathogenesis and the role of angiogenesis in the pathophysiological processes and treatments of both anomalies.

Port Wine Stain (PWS)

Port wine stain (PWS), also known as nevus flammeus, is a congenital, cutaneous vascular malformation which causes a pink to red to violet skin discoloration. PWS occurs in an estimated 3–5 children per 1000 live births and equally affects both genders and all races [2, 5]. There are no reports of a hereditary tendency for PWS or ways to predict or prevent PWS.

PWS can appear anywhere on the body, but most malformations occur on the face and neck. The negative reaction of others to a "marked" person adversely influences the personality development of virtually all patients. Studies have documented that PWS patients have lower self-esteem and problems with interpersonal relationships [6–8]. PWS is a progressive malformation, and there is no spontaneous involution. In childhood, PWS is a flat red macule (Fig. 8.1a), but lesions tend to darken progressively to purple and, by middle age, often become raised as a result of the development of skin thickening and vascular nodules. Hypertrophy of underlying soft tissue, which occurs in approximately two-thirds of lesions, further disfigures the facial features of many patients (Fig. 8.1b) [9, 10]. In conclusion, PWS is a clinically significant disease in the majority of patients with potentially devastating psychological and physiological complications. Moreover, PWS may be a part of a larger disorder or syndrome such as Sturge-Weber, Klippel-Trenaunay and Cobb syndromes, which require medical intervention of the underlying malformations in addition to treatment of the superficial PWS.

Histopathological studies of PWS show a normal epidermis overlying an abnormal plexus of dilated blood vessels located in the upper 0.8–1 mm of the dermis [11]. However, vessels throughout the entire skin thickness are abnormally dilated

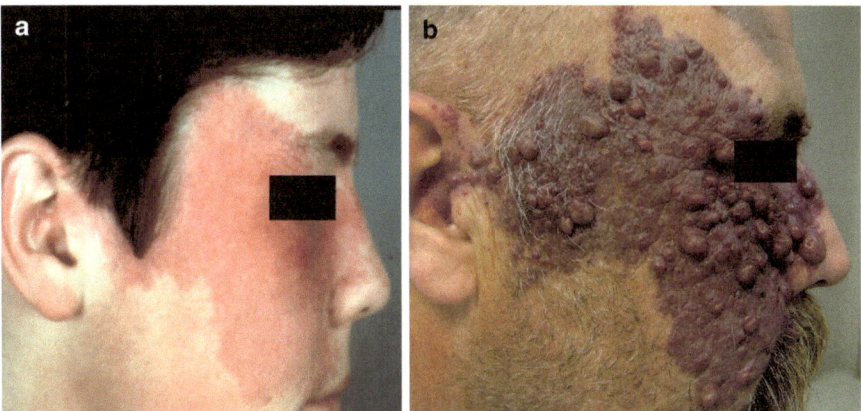

Fig. 8.1 (**a**) Adolescent male with PWS; (**b**) same male with PWS at 42 years of age. Note vascular nodules and soft tissue hypertrophy in (**b**) (Reprinted with permission from [9])

[11]. Electron microscopy exhibits vascular dilatations confined to postcapillary venules and thickening of the walls of the dilated venules [12, 13]. The endothelium of PWS blood vessels contains fenestrations and/or small gaps. Various alterations in the intervascular connective tissue have also been documented [13].

Pathogenesis of PWS

The pathogenesis of PWS remains incompletely understood. However, many lines of evidence have suggested that the nervous system is involved in the pathogenesis of PWS. Lesions on the face appear in the areas innervated by one or more branches of the trigeminal (V1, V2, V3) nerve. In a study of 310 PWS patients, 99 PWS were located on the area innervated by the second (V2) branch of the trigeminal nerve (32%), 128 in the combined first and second (V1, V2) branches (41%), 17 in the combined second and third (V2, V3) branches (5%), and 30 in all three branches (V1, V2, V3) (10%) [14]. The same study also showed that when PWS was involved in all three branches there was a significantly higher likelihood of eye and/or central nervous system complications.

Several studies have shown that there is a deficiency of nerve innervation to PWS vessels. Smoller et al. found, when staining the neural tissue with a S-100 antibody, that only 17% of the vessels in a PWS course with nerves, as compared to 89% in normal skin or hemangioma tissues [15]. Rydh et al. showed after staining the nerve fibers with antibodies against neuron specific enolase, calcitonin gene-related peptide and neurofilament, that pathologically dilated vessels in the middle and deep dermis had defective innervation with only single or no nerve fibers in their vicinity while other structures in the skin have a normal density of nerve fibers [16]. Selim et al. showed when staining the nerve fibers with an antibody against protein gene product 9.5 that nerve density was significantly decreased in all PWS sites as compared to normal skin [17]. Furthermore, when epinephrine was injected into the PWS dermis, the ectatic vessels did not constrict [18], suggesting that defects in proper tonic modulation received from the sympathetic nervous system leads to progressive ectasia of thin-walled vessels. Collectively, the lack of blood vessel innervation may contribute to the development of a PWS as a direct result of decreased tonus of the vessels and/or a loss of neuronal trophic factors.

Treatment of PWS

Historical treatments for PWS included skin grafting, ionizing radiation, dermabrasion, cryosurgery, and electrotherapy. Clinical results were unsatisfactory due to cosmetically unacceptable scarring post-treatment. The current treatment of choice for PWS is pulsed dye laser (PDL) therapy which is based on the theory of selective photothermolysis. This theory describes a method to selectively destroy subsurface-targets without inducing thermal damage in adjacent normal tissue [19]. To achieve this goal, a proper wavelength that is absorbed preferentially by a chromophore in the target, such as hemoglobin, should be chosen. To limit the amount of heat diffusing into the surrounding tissue during light exposure, the duration of laser irradiation should be on the order of the target's thermal relaxation time which is defined as the time required for the target to cool to one half of its peak temperature immediately after laser irradiation.

The first generation of PDL had a wavelength of 577 nm and pulse duration of 300 μs which was shown to cause selective vascular destruction in PWS skin without evidence of scarring [20]. A change in wavelength from 577 to 585 nm resulted in deeper penetration of the laser light and deeper blood vessel injury which is required for adult PWS treatment [21]. The incorporation of the dynamic cooling device into the PDL allows selective cooling of the epidermis, which is prone to injury due to light absorption by melanin, while leaving the temperature of the PWS blood vessels unchanged [22]. Dynamic skin cooling has permitted the use of higher light dosages to expedite PWS lesion clearance without producing complications such as dyspigmentation or scarring [23].

Despite the advancement in PDL and skin cooling techniques, complete PWS clearance is rarely achieved in the majority of cases even after multiple PDL treatments. Van der Horst et al. treated 89 patients with PWS aged from infancy to 31 years using the PDL [24]. The average reduction in PWS color was only 40%, and no patients had 100% clearance of their PWS after 5 treatments. In a study by Yohn et al. on 74 adult patients treated using the PDL, only 36.5% achieved 50% clearing, and no patients had 100% clearance of their PWS after 3–16 treatments [25]. A recent review by Lanigan and Taibjee concluded that "it remains difficult to eradicate PWS fully with our current armory of lasers and noncoherent light sources" [26].

Many factors contribute to incomplete PWS blanching. Epidermal melanin limits the light dosage that can be safely applied and reduces light delivery to targeted PWS vessels. When the PWS blood vessels are too small or too large, heat cannot be confined to or fill the entire lumen [27–29]. Regrowth and reperfusion of photo-coagulated blood vessels can cause PWS redarkening or treatment failure [30, 31]. We believe that the regrowth and reperfusion of blood vessels post-PDL treatment is a critical barrier to achieving an adequate PWS therapeutic outcome. As shown in Fig. 8.2, PDL resulted in intense purpura with histological documentation of vascular wall necrosis. However, the laser-induced wound healing response to PDL treatment often results in regrowth and reperfusion of PWS blood vessels within 1 month after laser exposure. As stated by Phung et al. [31], "the laser does what it

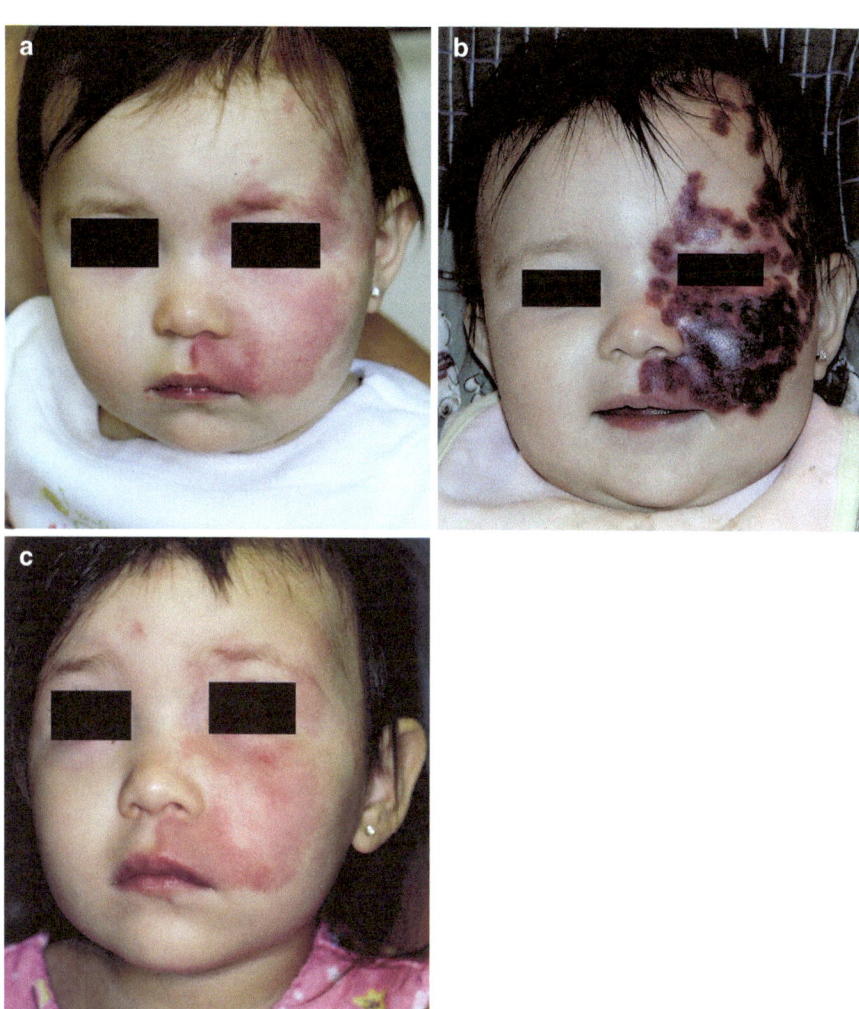

Fig. 8.2 (**a**), PWS before PDL treatment; (**b**), 2 days after treatment; (**c**), 1 year after PDL. Despite intense purpuric response induced by PDL treatment, the PWS blood vessels have reformed (Reprinted with permission from [31])

is supposed to do, namely, cause blood vessel wall necrosis. Regrettably, the body also does what it is supposed to do, namely, repair the laser-induced damage."

Angiogenesis and Vasculogenesis After PDL-Treatment

PDL treatment of PWS causes intense, acute damage to blood vessels [31, 32]. The skin's normal wound healing response detects hypoxia and initiates appropriate defense mechanisms, such as angiogenesis. The PDL-induced local hypoxia leads to upregulation of hypoxia-inducible factor-1alpha (HIF-1α), a master modulator for hypoxic response [33, 34] and vascular endothelial growth factor (VEGF) [33, 34], which subsequently activates many angiogenic signaling pathways and ultimately results in the regrowth and reperfusion of PWS blood vessels.

HIF-1α is known to control the expression of hundreds of genes involved in angiogenesis, inflammation, bioenergetics, proliferation, motility and apoptosis [35, 36]. As the key angiogenic molecule acting in response to oxygen concentration, HIF-1α is regulated at multiple levels in response to hypoxia. First, HIF-1α mRNA expression increases under hypoxia or ischemia. Many studies have shown that HIF-1α mRNA increases in response to hypoxia in rodents [37–40] and humans [41, 42]. Furthermore, the stabilization of HIF-1α mRNA may also contribute to the sustained increase of its mRNA [37]. Second, HIF-1α protein is synthesized and accumulated as a result of hypoxia stimulation. Hypoxia activates the mammalian target of rapamycin (mTOR) signaling pathway that plays a very important role in stimulation of the synthesis of HIF-1α protein and its transcriptional activities [36, 43]. HIF-1α has been shown as the downstream target of mTOR with an mTOR signaling motif located in its N terminus, which can interact with the regulatory associated protein of mTOR (Raptor) [43]. This pathway affects the translational levels of HIF-1α and serves as an amplifier for maximal expression of HIF-1α rather than the essential trigger for its activation [43].

The mRNA and protein levels of HIF-1α are significantly upregulated in animal skin irradiated by PDL as compared to normal skin [44]. In a hamster model, when the blood vessels are destroyed by laser [32, 44], the hypoxia induced by laser exposure is very severe and persistent for days until the vessels are fully reformed and reperfused. Thus, the increase of HIF-1α protein levels after laser treatment may be the result of both an increase in its mRNA level and translation rate. Furthermore, other angiogenic related biological processes, such as wound healing, defense and inflammatory responses, may also contribute to the increase in HIF-1α protein and mRNA levels in response to laser irradiation.

VEGF is the growth factor that plays a predominant role in angiogenesis pathways. VEGF can activate the vascular endothelial growth factor receptor 2 (VEGFR-2) which can then render the full range of VEGF responses such as endothelial cell proliferation, migration and formation of vascular tubulin [45, 46]. VEGF and HIF-1α can be upregulated reciprocally through angiogenesis pathways. VEGF is one of the downstream targets of HIF-1α. Hypoxia-activated-HIF-1α can translocate into the nucleus and directly bind to the hypoxia response element of the

VEGF promoter and activate its transcription, thus leading to an increase in VEGF mRNA levels [43, 47–49]. Alternatively, VEGF can increase HIF-1α mRNA translation into protein via phosphoinositide 3-kinase (PI3K) /AKT signaling [48, 50].

Both skin mRNA and protein levels of VEGF have been shown to increase significantly in a hamster animal model post-PDL exposure as compared to non-irradiated control skin [44], indicating an active role of VEGF in the angiogenesis process induced by laser irradiation. As the receptor of VEGF, which initiates the angiogenesis pathway, the protein level of VEGFR-2 is upregulated in laser-treated hamster skin as compared to non-irradiated control skin [51]. The 70 kDa ribosomal S6 kinase (S6) and AKT, the two main downstream molecules of VEGF, demonstrate an increase in their phosphorylation levels after PDL exposure [44], which suggests that the PIK3/AKT/mTOR pathway is activated through VEGF/VEGFR-2 signaling.

A schematic of the angiogenesis pathways in skin post-PDL exposure is outlined in Fig. 8.3. Briefly, PDL-induced hypoxia stabilizes and translocates HIF-1α into the nucleus as the initial step to trigger angiogenesis pathways. HIF-1α can bind to the hypoxia response element on promoters of many angiogenic genes, thus facilitating their transcription. These angiogenic growth

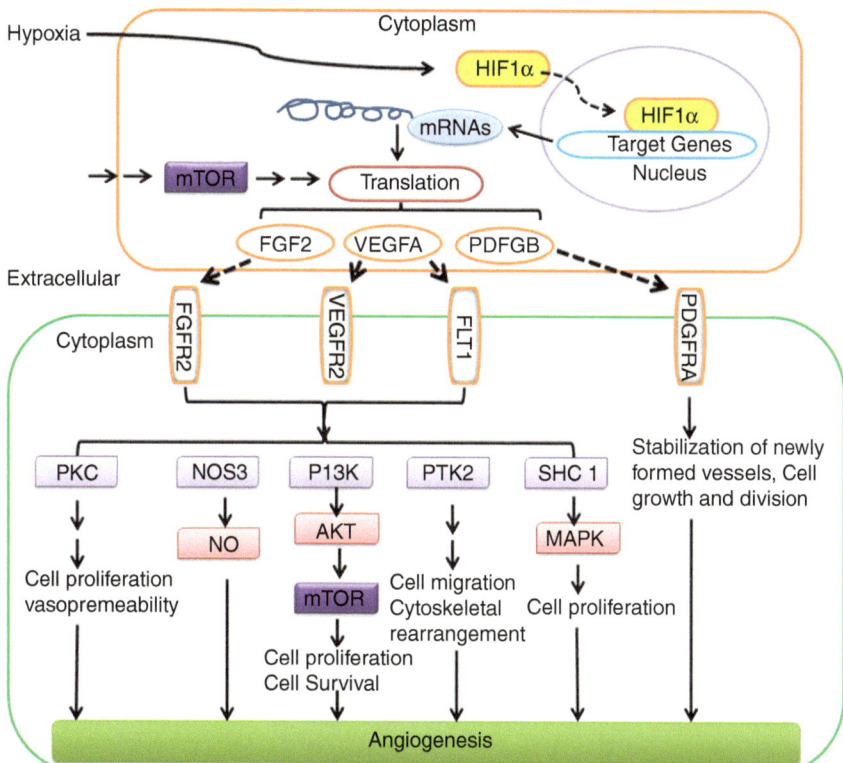

Fig. 8.3 A schematic of angiogenesis pathways activated by PDL exposure

factors, such as VEGF, fibroblast growth factor 2 (FGF2) and platelet-derived growth factor beta polypeptide (PDGFB), are regulated by HIF-1α at the transcriptional level and mTOR/S6 kinase signaling at the translational level. Ultimately, these factors are secreted into the extracelluar space between cells. These secreted growth factors bind to and activate their receptors, such as VEGFR2, FMS-like tyrosine kinase 1 (FLT1), fibroblast growth factor receptor 2 (FGFR2) and PDGF receptor, alpha polypeptide (PDGFRA), on adjacent cells. Activation of these receptors leads to the activation of multiple signaling pathways in adjacent cells, such as protein kinase C (PKC), endothelial nitric oxide synthase 3 (NOS3), PI3K/AKT, protein tyrosine kinase 2 (PTK2), SHC transforming protein 1 (SHC1)/mitogen-activated protein kinase (MAPK). These signaling pathways play important roles in cell proliferation, survival, migration, cytoskeletal rearrangement and blood vessel stabilization, which ultimately contribute to angiogenesis (Fig. 8.3).

In addition to angiogenesis, vasculogenesis may also be involved in regrowth and reperfusion of photocoagulated blood vessels. Recent evidence has shown that endothelial stem cells have been recruited into skin sites where blood vessel were photocoagulated [52], suggesting the possible role of vasculogenesis in the regrowth and reperfusion of blood vessels. Circulating endothelial stem cells are characterized by the expression of the cluster of differentiation 133 (CD133) [53] while mesenchymal stem cells are characterized by the expression of the cluster of differentiation 166 (CD166) [54]. After human skin is exposed to PDL, the stem cell marker nestin is strongly expressed in the proliferating endothelial cells but not CD133 or CD166 [52]. Nestin-expressing stem cells are primarily located in the hair follicular bulge region and contribute to the growth of new vessels in injured skin [55]. These results together suggest dermal follicular-derived, rather than bone marrow-derived, endothelial stem cells are locally recruited for the regrowth and reperfusion of PDL-injured blood vessels. However, the stem cell marker nestin is also upregulated in proliferating endothelial cells in human tumors [56, 57] and in activated endothelial cells in inflammation [58]; thus, additional work is needed to investigate the possible role of vasculogenesis during regrowth and reperfusion of PDL-injured skin blood vessels.

Anti-angiogenic Therapy for PWS Treatment

Presently, PDL treatment for PWS is inadequate to achieve complete lesion blanching due to regrowth and reperfusion of photocoagulated PWS blood vessels. In the pathophysiological process of PWS blood vessels regrowth and reperfusion, activation of angiogenesis pathways plays a major role. Thus, anti-angiogenic therapeutic strategies combined with PDL may potentially enhance PWS therapeutic outcome. Many anti-angiogenic drugs have been developed to target different signaling pathways in angiogenesis and have been approved by the US Food and Drug Administration for treating certain cancers [59]. However, only angiogenesis inhibitors without serious side effects should be used to treat PWS patients. One such compound is rapamycin (RPM) which has a long history of human use as an immunosuppressant with a relatively low side effect profile [60].

RPM can inhibit mTOR activity by forming a complex with FK-binding protein 12 and then binding to mTOR directly [61–63]. RPM has been used: (1) for immunosuppression in renal transplantation subjects [64]; (2) as anti-cancer therapy due to inhibition of tumor cell survival and angiogenesis [61, 65, 66]; and (3) for the treatment of hypervascular anomalies including angiomyolipomas [67–70] and many skin diseases, including Kaposi's sarcoma [42, 71, 72], psoriasis [73] and angiofibromas [74].

A preclinical animal study has been conducted to show the feasibility of antiangiogenic therapy for PWS treatment. The animal model used in this study is the dorsal window chamber installed on Golden Syrian hamsters. The model consists of a lengthwise fold of dorsal skin held with two titanium frames. One layer of skin within the frame's observation window was cut to expose the subdermal blood vessels in the underlying intact skin. This model permits in vivo visualization and irradiation of the subdermal blood vessels.

Laser irradiation was performed on the subdermal side of the skin through the window glass. Blood vessels were irradiated with a frequency-doubled Nd:YAG laser (532 nm wavelength). The pulse duration was 1 ms and the radiant exposure varied from 3 to 5 J/cm^2. The laser spot size was 2 mm (circles in Fig. 8.4). The number of pulses varied from 1 to 5 and the pulse repetition rate was 20 Hz.

Topical RPM was applied onto the epidermal side of the skin in the window chamber immediately after laser irradiation and daily thereafter for 14 days. The RPM formula contained 1% RPM powder dissolved in 5% benzyl alcohol and thoroughly mixed with a skin penetration enhancer and an ointment base (Conrex Pharmaceuticals, Newtown Square, PA).

To document the structural and functional changes of blood vessels induced by laser irradiation or drug intervention, digital color photos and laser speckle images (LSI) of the windows were acquired prior to, shortly after laser irradiation, and daily thereafter for 2 weeks. LSI was used to determine blood flow dynamics in the window [75].

When animal skin was exposed to laser, acute vessel injury with a reduction or stoppage in blood flow was observed immediately after exposure. However, regrowth and reperfusion of the blood vessels were completed by day 14 when laser was used alone, a process that is normally observed within 10 days post-laser irradiation (Fig. 8.4 – Laser Alone). In contrast, there were little regrowth and reperfusion of blood vessels after light-induced blood vessel coagulation in conjunction with daily topical application of RPM (Fig. 8.4 – Laser+RPM). Even after RPM was discontinued for 21 days, only 20% regrowth and reperfusion was observed in the skin microvasculature during this period [31, 32].

Our recent study showed that the VEGF/AKT/mTOR pathway activated by PDL irradiation can be suppressed by RPM [76]. In an animal model, topical application of RPM suppressed the PDL-induced increase in mRNA and protein levels of VEGF on day 3 post-PDL exposure. The upregulation of phosphorylation levels of S6 (Ser411) and AKT (Ser473) induced by PDL exposure was also suppressed with

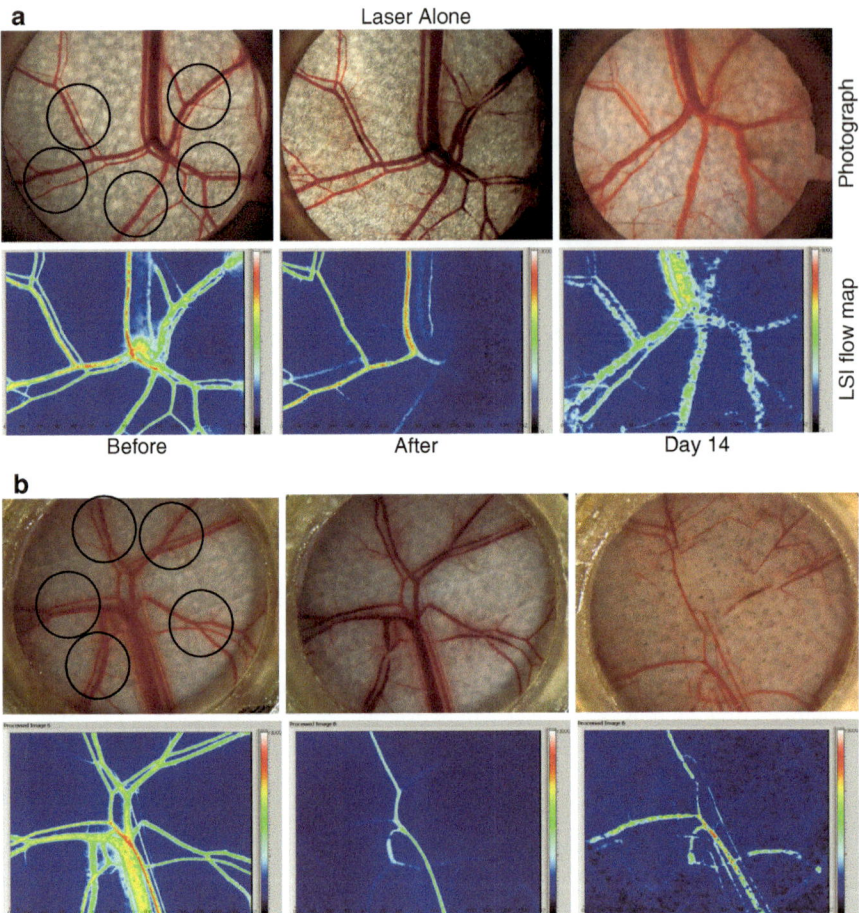

Fig. 8.4 (**a**), (*Laser alone*) Photos of the subdermal side of the window chamber before and after Laser alone treatment and 14 days later. At Day 14, blood vessel regrowth was observed. (**b**), (Laser+RPM) Laser plus 1% topical RPM treatment show little blood vessel regrowth and reperfusion 14 days after laser irradiation (Reprinted with permission from [31, 32])

RPM, which is consistent with studies with other animal and disease models [77, 78]. One possible mechanism to inhibit VEGF by topical RPM is that the suppression of mTOR with RPM downregulates HIF-1α levels and thus decreases its transcriptional activity to the VEGF promoter [61, 79–82].

Similar to VEGF, the PDL-induced increase in mRNA and protein levels of HIF-1α can also be suppressed by topical application of RPM [76]. RPM has been demonstrated to downregulate hypoxia-induced HIF-1α protein and mRNA levels in many other tissues and models [43, 79–81, 83]. The proposed mechanism is that RPM can directly suppress the translation process of HIF-1α through inhibition of mTOR signaling and modulate HIF-1α activity via a Von Hippel-Lindau-independent mechanism, but RPM does not affect the stability of HIF-1α protein [43].

A pilot clinical study has been conducted to determine the safety and efficacy of combined oral RPM and PDL therapy on PWS test sites in comparison to standard PDL therapy [84]. The hypothesis is that PDL can cause PWS blood vessel injury and RPM can prevent blood vessels regrowth and reperfusion after laser therapy which will improve PWS lesion blanching response.

An adult male PWS patient with a lesion involving his left chest was recruited. Three test sites with a diameter of 2.5 cm were selected (Fig. 8.5a) and treated by PDL alone as controls. One month after PDL alone exposure, the subject was given 2 mg RPM per day orally. On the seventh day after daily RPM intake, three additional test sites were then treated by PDL using the same parameters as the PDL alone test sites. The subject continued taking oral RPM for 4 weeks after the second laser exposure.

Photographs of the test sites at baseline, 6 weeks, 8 and 13 months are shown in Fig. 8.5a, b, c, d. On the PDL alone test site, some blanching was observed at 6 weeks after treatment (Fig. 8.5b). However, the test sites progressively darkened to almost unidentifiable at 8 and 13 months (Fig. 8.5c, d). In contrast, the test sites treated with the combined oral RPM and PDL therapy had better blanching responses as compared to PDL alone at 6 weeks after treatment (Fig. 8.5b). Even more impressively, the blanching of the test sites treated with the combined therapy has been maintained long-term for more than 13 months after treatment (Fig. 8.5c, d).

No abnormal wound healing, skin texture change and dyspigmentation was observed on any test site. Blood and urine test results at 2 and 4 weeks after the second laser treatment were within normal limits (trace protein noted on urinalysis.)

In summary, PWS is a congenital vascular malformation of skin with development of progressive blood vessel dilation within the lesion. A defect in nervous innervation to PWS blood vessels has been proposed to contribute to the pathogenesis of PWS. PDL treatment of PWS is inadequate to achieve complete lesion blanching due to regrowth and reperfusion of PWS blood vessels after PDL treatment. Angiogenesis pathways play critical roles in the pathophysiological process

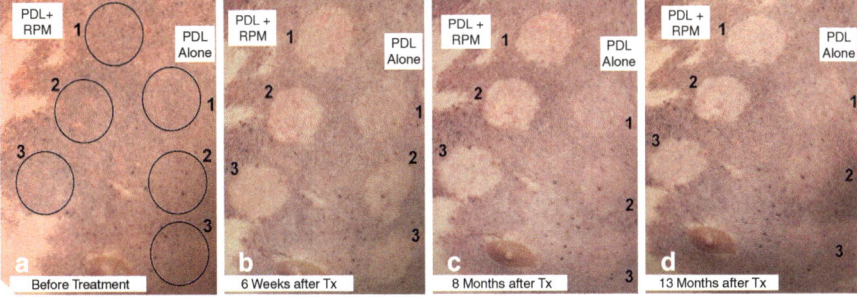

Fig. 8.5 PDL alone vs. oral RPM + PDL. Blanching responses by test sites and treatment: (**a**) before treatment; (**b**) 6 weeks after treatment; (**c**) 8 months after treatment; and (**d**) 13 months after treatment (Reprinted with permission from [84])

of regrowth and reperfusion of PWS blood vessels after PDL exposure. Multiple signaling pathways, including VEGF, FGF2 and PDGFB, are activated in response to PDL exposure. Thus, anti-angiogenic therapy combined with PDL should be considered as the future focus on new therapeutic strategies for PWS. One anti-angiogenic drug, RPM, can efficiently suppress the VEGF/PI3K/AKT/mTOR pathway and inhibit reperfusion of blood vessels post-PDL exposure in an animal model and PWS patients.

Infantile Hemangioma (IH)

Infantile hemangiomas (IH) are the most common tumors of infancy and occur in 4–5% of infants by 1 year of age. The majority of lesions are noted within the first few weeks of life [85]. For most children, the lesions are small and take on an uncomplicated course, but some hemangiomas grow dramatically so as to destroy tissue, impair function, or threaten life. A unique and defining feature of infantile hemangiomas is their remarkably predictable biologic behavior: a rapid proliferating phase followed by a slow spontaneous involution characterized by apoptosis and disappearance of capillaries with replacement by loose fibrofatty tissue. In the past decade, there have been immense advances in the pathogenesis of hemangiomas, providing us with insight on treatment and stimulating vascular regression.

Historical Perspective of Hemangiomas

The first theory on vascular tumors was developed in the 1950s, when light microscopy of IH revealed abnormal endothelia with cells forming poorly organized buds and irregular vascular spaces. It was postulated that IH developed from islands of angioblastic mesenchyma that were isolated from systemic vasculature during fetal development [86]. In the past few decades, new histopathologic techniques at the molecular and cellular level have significantly improved our understanding of these tumors.

The following review will discuss these findings and theories on the pathogenesis of IH. Several hypotheses have been proposed to explain their pathogenesis, but no single theory accounts for all of their features. Our current understanding of IH suggests that the pathogenesis is multifactorial, and that multiple genes, in addition to local effects, play a role in the development, growth and involution of IH.

Pathophysiology and Life Cycle of Infantile Hemangiomas

Infantile hemangiomas represent localized or regional areas of abnormal vascular development and proliferation. Histopathologic evaluation of tissue reveals characteristic findings in each phase of the life cycle.

The proliferating phase is characterized by the rapid proliferation of primitive cells and occurs during the first few weeks after birth to the end of infancy. Microscopically, IH demonstrate increased endothelial cellularity, formation of syncytial masses without a defined vascular architecture, proliferating endothelial cells and pericytes that focally form lumina containing red cells (Fig. 8.6) [87]. The endothelial and interstitial cells strongly express a marker of proliferation, MIB1. The number of cells in mitosis greatly exceeds the apoptotic cells and mitotic activity is easily observed in the proliferative phase with apoptosis less frequently detected. CD31+ endothelial cells are clonal and express a particular phenotype [88]: indoleamine 2,3 dioxygenase (IDO), LYVE-1, merosin, CCR6, glucose transporter (GLUT-1), antigen Lewis Y (Ley), and antigen FcRII (CD32). It has also been observed that hematopoietic cells of the myeloid lineage constitute a significant portion of the cells found in hemangiomas, particularly in the proliferative phase. Myeloid cells appear in large numbers during the proliferative phase and participate in angiogenesis through secretion of pro-angiogenic factors [89].

Spontaneous involution typically commences around 1 year of age and into early childhood. During the involution phase, the endothelial cells express caspases, which are known markers of apoptosis [90]. Light microscopy shows apoptotic bodies and increased number of mast cells are present and the endothelium begins to flatten, accompanied by enlargement of the lumen. Mitotic activity ceases

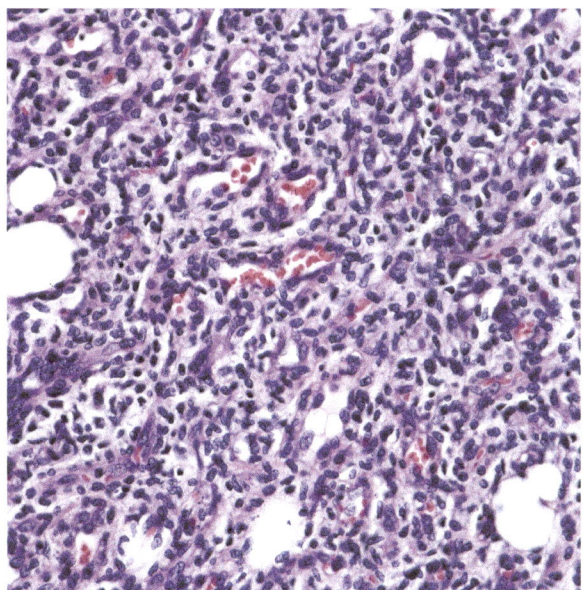

Fig. 8.6 Note the prominent spindle-shaped pericytes in aggregates. The endothelial spaces are scattered amidst these aggregates, and exhibit plump luminal cells. Note the numerous mitoses represented by dark oval, round, and rectangular-shaped structures. There are scattered mast cells and lymphocytes throughout the cellular population

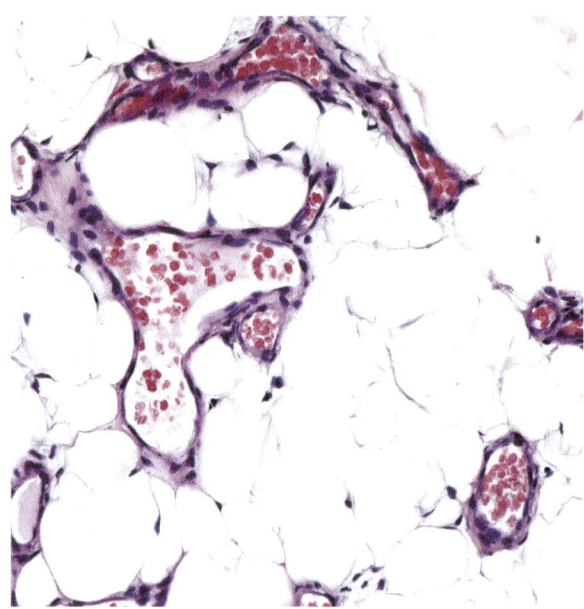

Fig. 8.7 As involution proceeds, the areas of endothelial cell proliferation are replaced by islands of stroma and adipocytes. The latest stages of involution exhibit fibro-adipose zones with only a few large vessels as any evidence of a prior vascular lesion at the site

and apoptotic cells are easily observed. In addition, a diffuse lymphocytic infiltrate with CD8+ T cytotoxic activity markers is also noted with positive granzyme B expression. This stage corresponds to an increase in the expression of markers of maturation and activation of endothelial cells such as HLA-DR and ICAM-1 (CD54) [91]. As involution proceeds, fibroadipose tissue increases and fills the vessels both within and between lobules (Fig. 8.7) [87, 91]. The origin of the adipocytes has been suggested to be derived from differentiated descendants of the primitive cells present in the proliferating phase and it has been shown that hemangioma stem cells are capable of differentiation into not only endothelial cells, but also adipocytes [92].

Angiogenesis and Vasculogenesis

Infantile hemangiomas are the result of the rapid development of blood vessels. The growth and involution of IH are unique in their lifecycle of proliferation and involution, and differ from other vascular anomalies, which do not regress over time. Blood vessels develop in vivo from two distinct processes: angiogenesis and vasculogenesis. Postnatal vasculogenesis is relatively uncommon and only occurs in specific circumstances, such as wound healing, placental formation, tumor growth and diseases of the eye [93]. Studies have shown that both angiogenesis and vasculogenesis participate in the formation of blood vessels, however more recent studies suggest that vasculogenesis may have a more important role in the development of IH.

Supporting the theory of angiogenesis is the detection of angiogenic factors such as bFGF and VEGF within the tumor, and up-regulation of angiogenesis-related integrin receptors in proliferating but not involuting IH [89, 94]. VEGF has been implicated in angiogenesis because it specifically induces proliferation of endothelial cells and results in increased vascular permeability. It has been observed that the expression of VEGFR1 in hemangioma endothelial cells and protein levels are abnormally low compared with different control endothelial cells. These low levels of VEGFR1 expression are associated with VEGF-induced activation of VEGFR2 and activation of downstream signaling pathways, which lead to stimulation of angiogenesis. Nuclear factor activated T-cells (NFAT) targets the VEGFR1 gene, resulting in its transcription in endothelial cells; suppression of NFAT increasing VEGF levels [95].

Notch family members have also recently been found to play a role in vascular development during tumor angiogenesis. The pattern of Notch gene expression has been shown to parallel the progression from immature cells to endothelial-lined vascular channels that characterizes the growth and involution of IH [96]. Notch3 was found to be expressed in hemangioma-derived stem cells but not in hemangioma-derived endothelial cells. This finding indicates that Notch3 was associated with proliferation, while increased expression of endothelial-associated Notch proteins Notch1, Notch4 and Jagged-1 was associated with maturation and involution.

More recently, studies have demonstrated that IH may arise from the process of vasculogenesis [97]. This theory suggests that IH may be derived from undifferentiated stem cells or progenitor cells from the placenta or bone marrow [95]. Hemangioma-derived endothelial cells (HemECs) were found to express many of the features of human endothelial cells and common endothelial markers. These cells exhibit clonality and increased rates of proliferation, adhesion and migration in response to endostatin, which normally inhibits migration and growth of mature endothelial cells [98]. These findings suggest that hemangiomas may result from a defect in endothelial differentiation or maturation. Hemangioma-derived endothelial progenitor cells (HemEPCs), a precursor of HemECs, have also been isolated from hemangiomas in the proliferating phase and found to co-express the human stem cell marker CD133 and endothelial cell markers and enhanced migration in response to endostatin. Endothelial progenitor cells (EPC) express HIF1α which in turn promotes local production of VEGF [99]. However, when implanted into immunodeficient mice, EPC was found to be incapable of new blood vessel formation [100]. This led to a search and identification of hemangioma-derived stem cell (HemSC), a multipotent progenitor-like cell that expresses CD90, a mesenchymal cell marker. These cells exhibit clonality and increased rates of proliferation and when implanted into immunodeficient mice, are capable of forming GLUT-1 positive hemangioma-like blood vessels, that subsequently decline and are replaced by adipocytes [92].

Theories of Hemangioma-Genesis and Involution

Placenta Theory

In recent years, there has been increasing evidence suggesting that the placenta is closely related to IH. It has been observed that the natural progression of IH parallels that of the placenta with proliferation in early gestation and stabilization thereafter. GLUT-1 was the first placental marker identified in IH and has become a hallmark histological tool in distinguishing these tumors from other vascular anomalies, in that it is a specific feature of IH during all phases of progression, and was not found in other vascular malformations [101]. In addition to GLUT-1, there is a distinct constellation of tissue-specific markers uniquely co-expressed by IH and placental microvessels, namely FcγRII, LeY and merosin. Other markers including insulin growth factor 2 (IGF2), type II 17-hydroxysteroid dehydrogenase (17HSDb2), tissue factor pathway inhibitor 2 (TFPI-2), type III iodothyronine deiodinase [102] and IDO have been discovered in recent years implying a unique relationship between the placenta and IH [103].

Further support of the placental origin is provided by results of a study using large-scale genomic analysis [104]. Cluster analysis showed that placenta and IH are as similar as normal lung and lung tumors, raising the interesting possibility of viewing the placenta as "tumor" and the hemangioma as "metastasis" [105]. When comparisons were restricted to genes with known expression in endothelial cells, the similarities were even greater; IH was more similar to placental samples than placental samples were to each other. A study by Barnes showed that gene expression of 21 endothelial-associated genes found high correlation coefficient for all IH-placental pairs [104].

Epidemiologic studies also support the placental IH relationship. It has been observed that IH are more prevalent in infants whose mothers underwent chorionic villus sampling. Placental complications such as placenta previa and preeclampsia, infants with premature birth, and lower birth weight are all associated with a higher incidence of the tumor [106, 107]. Trauma from placental complications and chorionic villus sampling may increase the number of placental cells released into the circulation and increase the likelihood of embolization of trophoblasts to fetal vascular sites. One study showed that infants of mothers who underwent chorionic villus sampling had a 10-fold greater incidence of hemangiomas compared with those who did not undergo this procedure [108, 109]. A more recent study, however, did not corroborate this association [107], with another study showing that all hemangioma endothelial cells matched the genotype of the child and not the maternal genotype [110].

Hypoxia Theory

Infantile hemangiomas often exhibit an initial blanched appearance, thought of as a "precursor" area of pallor that precedes the proliferative lesion [111]. The tissue associated with the pallor undergoes a hypoxic insult sensed by cells, which respond by modifying gene expression [112]. These modifications can enhance the ability of the cell to survive low oxygen conditions as well as induce expression of factors that promote the growth of new blood vessels. These transcriptional effects are mediated by HIF1-α, which are stabilized by hypoxia and increased estrogen levels, and upregulated in both the placenta and IH tissue [113, 114]. Of significance, GLUT-1 and insulin-like growth factor 2 (IGF-2) are present in IH at high levels, and are both under the control of HIF-1α and induced by hypoxia [115, 116]. A recent study observed increased GLUT-1 transcription, protein and activity levels in IH endothelial cells that were subjected to hypoxia [117]. As IGF-2 expression is induced under low oxygen conditions, this may explain the high levels of this factor observed during the phase of rapid IH proliferation [118].

Clonality of Infantile Hemangioma and the Progenitor Theory

Another hypothesis in the etiology of IH suggests that the basic defect is a genetic mutation of the endothelial cell, or its progenitor. Hemangioma-derived multipotential stem cells have been found to display a mesenchymal morphology, robust proliferation, and multilineage differentiation in vitro and form blood vessels with features of IH when injected into mice. This finding is unique to hemangioma-derived stem cells but not other cell lines in the tumor suggesting that hemangioma-derived stem cells are the cellular origin of IH [92]. The somatic mutation is thought to occur in a single endothelial progenitor, which then leads to dysregulation of the genes that control endothelial growth and subsequently alters patterns of gene expression in nearby cells to influence hemangiogenesis [119]. Chromosomal analysis has also demonstrated hemangioma endothelial cell clonality based on X chromosome inactivation patterns, which was not present in non-endothelial cells [98]. Further evidence is shown by X-linked human androgen receptor gene analysis (HUMARA) [120] which exploits the fact that in females, cells generally inactivate one copy of their X chromosome in a random fashion. When a tissue or sample of isolated cells shows a bias towards inactivation of one allele, it may indicate that these cells may have been derived from a single parent cell, which was shown in several studies of hemangioma endothelial cells and IH tissue [105, 119]. This is consistent with the possibility that these tumors are caused by somatic mutations in one or more genes regulating endothelial cell proliferation [98, 121]. Supporting this theory are cases of familial IH showing an autosomal dominant inheritance in the chromosomal region 5q31–33. Linkage analysis shows that this region contains three candidate genes involved in blood vessel growth: fibroblast growth factor receptor 4 (FGFR4), PDGF receptor (PDGFR)-beta, and VEGFR-3 (Flt-4) [121].

Further evidence is provided by studying lymphatic endothelial hyaluronan receptor-1 (LYVE-1), a specific marker for normal and tumor-associated lymphatic vessels that is expressed in IH during the proliferation and down-regulated during involution [122]. LYVE-1 has been shown to be a specific marker for the proliferating stage of IH since GLUT-1 is expressed in both phases. The demonstrated co-expression LYVE-1 and CD34 on hemangioma endothelial cells suggests that these cells have an immunophenotype similar to the cardinal vein during normal vascular development and supports the idea that hemangiomas arise from somatic mutation and clonal expansion of progenitor cells and that IH are arrested in the early developmental stage of vascular differentiation.

Passive and Active Involution Theory

One of the distinguishing features of IH compared with other vascular anomalies is the limited growth before self-involution. There have been two proposed theories to hemangioma involution. Apoptosis appears to be a major mechanism of cell death in the regressing tumor, but the events that trigger the apoptotic program have yet to be fully elucidated.

The first proposed mechanism is passive involution, where inherent properties of IH endothelial cells place limits on their proliferative lifespan. Similar to the clearly defined life cycle of placental tissue, it has been suggested that hemangioma cells also share this programmed lifespan subsequent to which programmed apoptosis will occur [123].

A second pathway involves active involution. It has been suggested IH cells carrying abnormal surface marker expression could be targeted by the immune system. One study showed a role for indoleamine 2,3-dioxygenase (IDO), an enzyme expressed in the proliferating IH in high levels but not in the involuting lesion. IDO acts as a T-cell toxin and prevents antigen presentation. IDO is highly expressed in the placenta and is thought to prevent rejection of the allogeneic fetus by catabolizing tryptophan, an amino acid crucial for the activation of T cells [124]. It has been postulated that the immune suppressive action of IDO might protect hemangioma cells from immune attack in the proliferating phase. In involution, antigen presentation is theoretically possible, leading to increased expression by CD8+ infiltrating cells that result in cell death.

Therapy Related to the Pathophysiology of Infantile Hemangioma

The current therapeutic modalities for the treatment of IH have shown varied response, and adverse effects of some therapeutic approaches limit their use (Table 8.1). Better understanding of the pathogenesis of IH may help to enable the development of more targeted therapeutic strategies. Several of the existing ones work by targeting different pathways of the IH.

Propranolol

Propranolol has become a widely accepted new therapy for complicated IH due to its relatively low side effect profile, rapid onset of action and favorable results. Propranolol was serendipitously discovered to be effective in the treatment of IH in 2008 and subsequently, numerous studies have reported success in clinically compromising cutaneous, orbital, visceral and airway IH as first-line therapy or in conjunction with systemic corticosteroids [130, 131]. Propranolol is thought to work by several mechanisms, including vasoconstriction, inhibition of angiogenesis and induction of apoptosis [132]. The early effects, which clinically reflect brightening and softening of the hemangioma within 1–3 days, are attributable to vasoconstriction of blood vessels due to decreased release of nitric oxide. Intermediate effects are due to inhibition of proangiogenic signals including VEGF, basic fibroblast growth factor and

Table 8.1 Therapies used in treatment of IH [125, 126]

Drug	Mechanism of action	Side effects
Triamcinolone Prednisonlone	Inhibit VEGF-induced angiogenesis Induction of endothelial cell apoptosis	(Systemic) Cushingoid appearance Adrenal suppression Hypertension Decreased growth Weight gain
Interferon alpha	Downregulation of VEGF expression leading to inhibition of angiogenesis [127]	Spastic diplegia [128] Leukopenia, neutropenia
Propranolol	Vasoconstriction Inhibition of angiogenesis Induction of apoptosis Reduction of renin activity	Hypotension Hypoglycemia Bradycardia Bronchospasm
Pulse dye laser	Selective absorption hemoglobin in vessels Damage to vessel wall, clot formation, vessel removal [19]	Ulceration Dyspigmentation
Bleomycin	Acts on S stage of DNA cell cycle to disrupt mitosis during cell proliferation Inhibition of neovascularization Inhibition of growth factor induced endothelial cell invasion, growth and migration Induction of endothelial cell apoptosis [129]	Edema Ulceration Dyspigmentation

HIF-1α, which arrest the growth of the tumor. Long-term effects of propranolol are characterized by induction of apoptosis in proliferating endothelial cells, resulting in tumor regression. It has also been proposed that angiotensin-converting enzyme and angiotensin receptor 2 play a role in IH. Angiotensin II has been found to cause secretion of VEGF from mesenchymal stem cells, proliferation of CD34+ cells and inhibition of mesenchymal stem cell differentiation into adipocytes [100]. These elevated levels of angiotensin II drive proliferation of vascular progenitor cell expression CD 34 within the hemangioma and prevent terminal differentiation of these cells into adipocytes. Beta-blockers may accelerate involution of IH by reducing renin activity, thereby lowering angiotensin I and angiotensin II levels.

Corticosteroids

Oral corticosteroid has been the mainstay therapy for complicated IH for many decades. The mechanism of action of corticosteroids was shown in a recent study that demonstrated that dexamethasone inhibited the vasculogenic potential of HemSC. Dexamethasone was found to specifically target the multipotential hemangioma stem cells by suppressing VEGF, leading to inhibition of vasculogenesis [133]. Corticosteroids have been shown to be more effective in the early proliferating phase of the IH than in the later proliferating phase [134], and may suggest that the response to treatment is determined by the ratio of immature stem cells to mature endothelial cells in the tumor [133].

Pulse Dye Laser

Pulse dye laser (PDL) has been shown to be an effective treatment for superficial hemangiomas and in patients with contraindications for systemic therapies or localized lesions, with one study showing that superficial IH treated with PDL showed reduction in redness and greater rate of clearance at 1 year [135]. PDL allows for targeted results, especially in anatomically or cosmetically sensitive areas and has been shown to decrease the proliferative phase and increase the rate of involution with the benefit of no systemic side effects [136]. When treatment was administered every 2–3 weeks and initiated early, it reduced the development of atrophy and telangiectasias by stunting the proliferative growth and expediting its resolution. In addition, PDL has been shown to increase production of dermal collagen and elastic fibers.

Conclusion

In the last 40 years, several important milestones have been reached in the study of vascular malformations. These include the seminal classification of Mulliken and Glowacki, the discovery of GLUT-1 and the resultant further understanding of molecular pathology of the lesions, the development and refinement of the lasers in the treatment of the lesions, and the various pharmacologic agents that have been introduced. In this chapter, we have discussed only two of the numerous vascular anomalies, namely the port wine stains and infantile hemangiomas. Our emphasis has been on a clear approach to clinical and pathological correlation, understanding pathogenesis, and an updated discussion of therapy in these lesions. While great strides have been made, in the last 15 years especially, they have only begun to open the door to a profound understanding of not only vascular anomalies, but also to the formation of blood vessels and their relationship to the nervous system in development.

References

1. Mulliken JB, Glowacki J. Hemangiomas and vascular malformations in infants and children: a classification based on endothelial characteristics. Plast Reconstr Surg. 1982;69(3): 412–22.
2. Jacobs AH, Walton RG. The incidence of birthmarks in the neonate. Pediatrics. 1976;58:218–22.
3. Mulliken JB, Young AR. Vascular birthmarks–hemangiomas and malformations. Philadelphia: W.B. Saunders Co.; 1988.
4. Pratt AG. Birthmarks in infants. Arch Derm Syphilol. 1953;67:302–5.
5. Alper JC, Holmes LB. The incidence and significance of birthmarks in a cohort of 4641 newborns. Pediatr Dermatol. 1986;1:58–68.
6. Kalick SM. Toward an interdisciplinary psychology of appearances. Psychiatry. 1978;41(3):243–53.
7. Heller A, Rafman S, Zvagulis I, Pless IB. Birth-defects and psychosocial adjustment. Am J Dis Child. 1985;139(3):257–63.
8. Malm M, Carlberg M. Port-wine stain – a surgical and psychological problem. Ann Plast Surg. 1988;20(6):512–6.
9. Minkis K, Geronemus RG, Hale EK. Port wine stain progression: a potential consequence of delayed and inadequate treatment? Lasers Surg Med. 2009;41(6):423–6.

10. Geronemus RG, Ashinoff R. The medical necessity of evaluation and treatment of port-wine stains. J Dermatol Surg Oncol. 1991;17(1):76–9.
11. Barsky SH, Rosen S, Geer DE, Noe JM. The nature and evolution of port wine stains: a computer-assisted study. J Invest Dermatol. 1980;74(3):154–7.
12. Braverman IM, Kehyen A. Ultrastructure and 3-dimensional reconstruction of several macular and papular telangiectases. J Invest Dermatol. 1983;81(6):489–97.
13. Schneider BV, Mitsuhashi Y, Schnyder UW. Ultrastructural observations in port wine stains. Arch Dermatol Res. 1988;280(6):338–45.
14. Tallman B, Tan OT, Morelli JG, Piepenbrink J, Stafford TJ, Trainor S, Weston WL. Location of port-wine stains and the likelihood of ophthalmic and/or central nervous system complications. Pediatrics. 1991;87(3):323–7.
15. Smoller BR, Rosen S. Port-wine stains. A disease of altered neural modulation of blood vessels? Arch Dermatol. 1986;122(2):177–9.
16. Rydh M, Malm M, Jernbeck J, Dalsgaard CJ. Ectatic blood vessels in port-wine stains lack innervation: possible role in pathogenesis. Plast Reconstr Surg. 1991;87(3):419–22.
17. Selim MM, Kelly KM, Nelson JS, Wendelschafer-Crabb G, Kennedy WR, Zelickson BD. Confocal microscopy study of nerves and blood vessels in untreated and treated port wine stains: preliminary observations. Dermatol Surg. 2004;30(6):892–7.
18. Rosen S, Smoller B. Pathogenesis of port wine stains. A new hypothesis. Med Hypotheses. 1987;22(4):365–8.
19. Anderson RR, Parrish JA. Selective photothermolysis – precise microsurgery by selective absorption of pulsed radiation. Science. 1983;220(4596):524–7.
20. Morelli JG, Tan OT, Garden J, Margolis R, Seki Y, Boll J, Carney JM, Anderson RR, Furumoto H, Parrish JA. Tunable dye laser (577 nm) treatment of port wine stains. Lasers Surg Med. 1986;6(1):94–9.
21. Tan OT, Morrison P, Kurban AK. 585-Nm for the treatment of port-wine stains. Plast Reconstr Surg. 1990;86(6):1112–7.
22. Nelson JS, Milner TE, Anvari B, Tanenbaum BS, Kimel S, Svaasand LO, Jacques SL. Dynamic epidermal cooling during pulsed laser treatment of port-wine stain: a new methodology with preliminary clinical evaluation. Arch Dermatol. 1995;131(6): 695–700.
23. Chang CJ, Nelson JS. Cryogen spray cooling and higher fluence pulsed dye laser treatment improve port-wine stain clearance while minimizing epidermal damage. Dermatol Surg. 1999;25(10):767–72.
24. van der Horst CMAM, Koster PHL, de Borgie CAJM, Bossuyt PMM, van Gemert MJC. Effect of the timing of treatment of port-wine stains with the flash-lamp-pumped pulsed dye-laser. New Engl J Med. 1998;338(15):1028–33.
25. Yohn JJ, Huff JC, Aeling JL, Walsh P, Morelli JG. Lesion size is a factor for determining the rate of port-wine stain clearing following pulsed dye laser treatment in adults. Cutis. 1997;59(5):267–70.
26. Lanigan SW, Taibjee SM. Recent advances in laser treatment of port-wine stains. Brit J Dermatol. 2004;151(3):527–33.
27. Fiskerstrand EJ, Svaasand LO, Kopstad G, Dalaker M, Norvang LT, Volden G. Laser treatment of port wine stains: therapeutic outcome in relation to morphological parameters. Br J Dermatol. 1996;134(6):1039–43.
28. Hohenleutner U, Hilbert M, Wlotzke U, Landthaler M. Epidermal damage and limited coagulation depth with the flashlamp-pumped pulsed dye-laser – a histochemical-study. J Invest Dermatol. 1995;104(5):798–802.
29. Jia W, Choi B, Franco W, Lotfi J, Majaron B, Aguilar G, Nelson JS. Treatment of cutaneous vascular lesions using multiple-intermittent cryogen spurts and two-wavelength laser pulses: numerical and animal studies. Lasers Surg Med. 2007;39(6):494–503.
30. Huikeshoven M, Koster PHL, de Borgie C, Beek JF, van Gemert MJC, van der Horst C. Redarkening of port-wine stains 10 years after pulsed-dye-laser treatment. New Engl J Med. 2007;356(12):1235–40.

31. Phung TL, Oble DA, Jia W, Benjamin LE, Mihm Jr MC, Nelson JS. Can the wound healing response of human skin be modulated after laser treatment and the effects of exposure extended? Implications on the combined use of the pulsed dye laser and a topical angiogenesis inhibitor for treatment of port wine stain birthmarks. Lasers Surg Med. 2008;40(1):1–5.
32. Jia W, Sun V, Tran N, Choi B, Liu SW, Mihm Jr MC, Phung TL, Nelson JS. Long-term blood vessel removal with combined laser and topical rapamycin antiangiogenic therapy: implications for effective port wine stain treatment. Lasers Surg Med. 2010;42(2):105–12.
33. Coulon C, Georgiadou M, Roncal C, De Bock K, Langenberg T, Carmeliet P. From vessel sprouting to normalization: role of the prolyl hydroxylase domain protein/hypoxia-inducible factor oxygen-sensing machinery. Arterioscler Thromb Vasc Biol. 2010;30(12):2331–6.
34. Fong GH. Regulation of angiogenesis by oxygen sensing mechanisms. J Mol Med (Berl). 2009;87(6):549–60.
35. Pugh CW, Ratcliffe PJ. Regulation of angiogenesis by hypoxia: role of the HIF system. Nat Med. 2003;9(6):677–84.
36. Semenza GL. Hypoxia-inducible factors in physiology and medicine. Cell. 2012;148(3): 399–408.
37. Wang GL, Jiang BH, Rue EA, Semenza GL. Hypoxia-inducible factor 1 is a basic-helix-loop-helix-PAS heterodimer regulated by cellular O2 tension. Proc Natl Acad Sci U S A. 1995;92(12):5510–4.
38. Wiener CM, Booth G, Semenza GL. In vivo expression of mRNAs encoding hypoxia-inducible factor 1. Biochem Biophys Res Commun. 1996;225(2):485–8.
39. Palmer LA, Semenza GL, Stoler MH, Johns RA. Hypoxia induces type II NOS gene expression in pulmonary artery endothelial cells via HIF-1. Am J Physiol. 1998;274(2 Pt 1): L212–9.
40. Bergeron M, Yu AY, Solway KE, Semenza GL, Sharp FR. Induction of hypoxia-inducible factor-1 (HIF-1) and its target genes following focal ischaemia in rat brain. Eur J Neurosci. 1999;11(12):4159–70.
41. Pialoux V, Mounier R, Brown AD, Steinback CD, Rawling JM, Poulin MJ. Relationship between oxidative stress and HIF-1 alpha mRNA during sustained hypoxia in humans. Free Radic Biol Med. 2009;46(2):321–6.
42. Zmonarski SC, Boratynska M, Rabczynski J, Kazimierczak K, Klinger M. Regression of Kaposi's sarcoma in renal graft recipients after conversion to sirolimus treatment. Transplant Proc. 2005;37(2):964–6.
43. Land SC, Tee AR. Hypoxia-inducible factor 1alpha is regulated by the mammalian target of rapamycin (mTOR) via an mTOR signaling motif. J Biol Chem. 2007;282(28):20534–43.
44. Tan W, Jia W, Sun V, Mihm MC, Nelson JS. Topical rapamycin suppresses the angiogenesis pathways induced by pulsed dye laser: mechanisms of inhibition of regeneration and revascularization of photocoagulated blood vessels lasers in surgery and medicine. Lasers Surg Med. 2012;44(10):796–804.
45. Carmeliet P, Jain RK. Molecular mechanisms and clinical applications of angiogenesis. Nature. 2011;473(7347):298–307.
46. Koch S, Tugues S, Li X, Gualandi L, Claesson-Welsh L. Signal transduction by vascular endothelial growth factor receptors. Biochem J. 2011;437(2):169–83.
47. Sekiguchi Y, Zhang J, Patterson S, Liu L, Hamada C, Tomino Y, Margetts PJ. Rapamycin inhibits transforming growth factor beta induced peritoneal angiogenesis by blocking the secondary hypoxic response. J Cell Mol Med. 2012;16(8):12.
48. Semenza GL. HIF-1: using two hands to flip the angiogenic switch. Cancer Metastasis Rev. 2000;19(1–2):59–65.
49. Semenza GL. Vascular responses to hypoxia and ischemia. Arterioscler Thromb Vasc Biol. 2010;30(4):648–52.
50. Kilic E, Kilic U, Wang Y, Bassetti CL, Marti HH, Hermann DM. The phosphatidylinositol-3 kinase/Akt pathway mediates VEGF's neuroprotective activity and induces blood brain barrier permeability after focal cerebral ischemia. FASEB J. 2006;20(8):1185–7.

51. Tan W, Jia W, Sun V, Nelson JS. Rapamycin reverses the process of regeneration and revascularization of photocoagulated blood vessels in an animal model. American Society for Laser Medicine and Surgery Annual Conference, vol. 44. Kissimmee: Wiley; 2012. p. 39.
52. Loewe R, Oble DA, Valero T, Zukerberg L, Mihm Jr MC, Nelson JS. Stem cell marker upregulation in normal cutaneous vessels following pulsed-dye laser exposure and its abrogation by concurrent rapamycin administration: implications for treatment of port-wine stain birthmarks. J Cutan Pathol. 2010;37(Suppl 1):76–82.
53. Ribatti D. The involvement of endothelial progenitor cells in tumor angiogenesis. J Cell Mol Med. 2004;8(3):294–300.
54. Oswald J, Boxberger S, Jorgensen B, Feldmann S, Ehninger G, Bornhauser M, Werner C. Mesenchymal stem cells can be differentiated into endothelial cells in vitro. Stem Cells. 2004;22(3):377–84.
55. Amoh Y, Li L, Yang M, Moossa AR, Katsuoka K, Penman S, Hoffman RM. Nascent blood vessels in the skin arise from nestin-expressing hair-follicle cells. Proc Natl Acad Sci U S A. 2004;101(36):13291–5.
56. Shimizu T, Sugawara K, Tosaka M, Imai H, Hoya K, Takeuchi T, Sasaki T, Saito N. Nestin expression in vascular malformations: a novel marker for proliferative endothelium. Neurol Med Chir (Tokyo). 2006;46(3):111–7.
57. Sugawara K, Kurihara H, Negishi M, Saito N, Nakazato Y, Sasaki T, Takeuchi T. Nestin as a marker for proliferative endothelium in gliomas. Lab Invest. 2002;82(3):345–51.
58. Ishiwata T, Kudo M, Onda M, Fujii T, Teduka K, Suzuki T, Korc M, Naito Z. Defined localization of nestin-expressing cells in L-arginine-induced acute pancreatitis. Pancreas. 2006;32(4):360–8.
59. Oklu R, Walker TG, Wicky S, Hesketh R. Angiogenesis and current antiangiogenic strategies for the treatment of cancer. J Vasc Interv Radiol. 2010;21(12):1791–805.
60. Kahan BD, Rapamune USSG. Efficacy of sirolimus compared with azathioprine for reduction of acute renal allograft rejection: a randomised multicentre study. Lancet. 2000;356(9225):194–202.
61. Guba M, von Breitenbuch P, Steinbauer M, Koehl G, Flegel S, Hornung M, Bruns CJ, Zuelke C, Farkas S, Anthuber M, Jauch KW, Geissler EK. Rapamycin inhibits primary and metastatic tumor growth by antiangiogenesis: involvement of vascular endothelial growth factor. Nat Med. 2002;8(2):128–35.
62. Kwon YS, Hong HS, Kim JC, Shin JS, Son Y. Inhibitory effect of rapamycin on corneal neovascularization in vitro and in vivo. Invest Ophthalmol Vis Sci. 2005;46(2):454–60.
63. Huang S, Bjornsti MA, Houghton PJ. Rapamycins: mechanism of action and cellular resistance. Cancer Biol Ther. 2003;2(3):222–32.
64. Saunders RN, Metcalfe MS, Nicholson ML. Rapamycin in transplantation: a review of the evidence. Kidney Int. 2001;59(1):3–16.
65. Guertin DA, Sabatini DM. Defining the role of mTOR in cancer. Cancer Cell. 2007;12(1):9–22.
66. Law BK. Rapamycin: an anti-cancer immunosuppressant? Crit Rev Oncol Hematol. 2005;56(1):47–60.
67. Wienecke R, Fackler I, Linsenmaier U, Mayer K, Licht T, Kretzler M. Antitumoral activity of rapamycin in renal angiomyolipoma associated with tuberous sclerosis complex. Am J Kidney Dis. 2006;48(3):E27–9.
68. Herry I, Neukirch C, Debray MP, Mignon F, Crestani B. Dramatic effect of sirolimus on renal angiomyolipomas in a patient with tuberous sclerosis complex. Eur J Intern Med. 2007;18(1):76–7.
69. Morton JM, McLean C, Booth SS, Snell GI, Whitford HM. Regression of pulmonary lymphangioleiomyomatosis (PLAM)-associated retroperitoneal angiomyolipoma post-lung transplantation with rapamycin treatment. J Heart Lung Transplant. 2008;27(4):462–5.
70. Bissler JJ, McCormack FX, Young LR, Elwing JM, Chuck G, Leonard JM, Schmithorst VJ, Laor T, Brody AS, Bean J, Salisbury S, Franz DN. Sirolimus for angiomyolipoma in tuberous sclerosis complex or lymphangioleiomyomatosis. New Engl J Med. 2008;358(2):140–51.

71. Yilmaz R, Akoglu H, Yirkpantur A, Kilickap S, Arici M, Altun B, Aki T, Erdem Y, Yasavul U, Turgan C. A novel immunosuppressive agent, sirolimus, in the treatment of Kaposi's sarcoma in a renal transplant recipient. Ren Fail. 2007;29(1):103–5.

72. Stallone G, Schena A, Infante B, Di Paolo S, Loverre A, Maggio G, Ranieri E, Gesualdo L, Schena FP, Grandaliano G. Sirolimus for Kaposi's sarcoma in renal-transplant recipients. New Engl J Med. 2005;352(13):1317–23.

73. Ormerod AD, Shah SAA, Copeland P, Omar G, Winfield A. Treatment of psoriasis with topical sirolimus: preclinical development and a randomized, double-blind trial. Brit J Dermatol. 2005;152(4):758–64.

74. Haemel AK, O'Brian AL, Teng JM. Topical rapamycin a novel approach to facial angiofibromas in tuberous sclerosis. Arch Dermatol. 2010;146(7):715–8.

75. Choi B, Kang NM, Nelson JS. Laser speckle imaging for monitoring blood flow dynamics in the in vivo rodent dorsal skin fold model. Microvasc Res. 2004;68(2):143–6.

76. Tan W, Jia W, Sun V, Mihm MC, Nelson JS. Topical rapamycin suppresses the angiogenesis pathways induced by pulsed dye laser: mechanisms of inhibition of regeneration and revascularization of photocoagulated blood vessels. Laser Surg Med. 2012;44(10):796–804. in press.

77. Medici D, Olsen BR. Rapamycin inhibits proliferation of hemangioma endothelial cells by reducing HIF-1-dependent expression of VEGF. PLoS One. 2012;7(8):e42913.

78. Phung TL, Ziv K, Dabydeen D, Eyiah-Mensah G, Riveros M, Perruzzi C, Sun J, Monahan-Earley RA, Shiojima I, Nagy JA, Lin MI, Walsh K, Dvorak AM, Briscoe DM, Neeman M, Sessa WC, Dvorak HF, Benjamin LE. Pathological angiogenesis is induced by sustained Akt signaling and inhibited by rapamycin. Cancer Cell. 2006;10(2):159–70.

79. Chen H, Xiong T, Qu Y, Zhao F, Ferriero D, Mu D. mTOR activates hypoxia-inducible factor-1alpha and inhibits neuronal apoptosis in the developing rat brain during the early phase after hypoxia-ischemia. Neurosci Lett. 2012;507(2):118–23.

80. Sekiguchi Y, Zhang J, Patterson S, Liu L, Hamada C, Tomino Y, Margetts PJ. Rapamycin inhibits transforming growth factor beta induced peritoneal angiogenesis by blocking the secondary hypoxic response. J Cell Mol Med. 2011;16(8):1934–45.

81. Wang W, Jia WD, Xu GL, Wang ZH, Li JS, Ma JL, Ge YS, Xie SX, Yu JH. Antitumoral activity of rapamycin mediated through inhibition of HIF-1alpha and VEGF in hepatocellular carcinoma. Dig Dis Sci. 2009;54(10):2128–36.

82. Vuiblet V, Birembaut P, Francois A, Cordonnier C, Noel LH, Goujon JM, Paraf F, Machet MC, Girardot-Seguin S, Lebranchu Y, Rieu P. Sirolimus-based regimen is associated with decreased expression of glomerular vascular endothelial growth factor. Nephrol Dial Transplant. 2012;27(1):411–6.

83. Hudson CC, Liu M, Chiang GG, Otterness DM, Loomis DC, Kaper F, Giaccia AJ, Abraham RT. Regulation of hypoxia-inducible factor 1alpha expression and function by the mammalian target of rapamycin. Mol Cell Biol. 2002;22(20):7004–14.

84. Nelson JS, Jia W, Phung TL, Mihm Jr MC. Observations on enhanced port wine stain blanching induced by combined pulsed dye laser and rapamycin administration. Laser Surg Med. 2011;43(10):939–42.

85. Kilcline C, Frieden IJ. Infantile hemangiomas: how common are they? A systematic review of the medical literature. Pediatr Dermatol. 2008;25(2):168–73.

86. Innes FL. Classification of haemangiomata. Br J Plast Surg. 1953;6(2):76–7.

87. Lo K, Mihm M, Fay A. Current theories on the pathogenesis of infantile hemangioma. Semin Ophthalmol. 2009;24(3):172–7.

88. Yu Y, Flint AF, Mulliken JB, Wu JK, Bischoff J. Endothelial progenitor cells in infantile hemangioma. Blood. 2004;103(4):1373–5.

89. Ritter MR, Dorrell MI, Edmonds J, Friedlander SF, Friedlander M. Insulin-like growth factor 2 and potential regulators of hemangioma growth and involution identified by large-scale expression analysis. Proc Natl Acad Sci U S A. 2002;99(11):7455–60.

90. Razon MJ, Kraling BM, Mulliken JB, Bischoff J. Increased apoptosis coincides with onset of involution in infantile hemangioma. Microcirculation. 1998;5(2–3):189–95.

91. Leaute-Labreze C, Prey S, Ezzedine K. Infantile haemangioma: part I. Pathophysiology, epidemiology, clinical features, life cycle and associated structural abnormalities. J Eur Acad Dermatol Venereol. 2011;25(11):1245–53.
92. Khan ZA, Boscolo E, Picard A, Psutka S, Melero-Martin JM, Bartch TC, Mulliken JB, Bischoff J. Multipotential stem cells recapitulate human infantile hemangioma in immunodeficient mice. J Clin Invest. 2008;118(7):2592–9.
93. Chiller KG, Frieden IJ, Arbiser JL. Molecular pathogenesis of vascular anomalies: classification into three categories based upon clinical and biochemical characteristics. Lymphat Res Biol. 2003;1(4):267–81.
94. Takahashi K, Mulliken JB, Kozakewich HP, Rogers RA, Folkman J, Ezekowitz RA. Cellular markers that distinguish the phases of hemangioma during infancy and childhood. J Clin Invest. 1994;93(6):2357–64.
95. Jinnin M, Medici D, Park L, Limaye N, Liu Y, Boscolo E, Bischoff J, Vikkula M, Boye E, Olsen BR. Suppressed NFAT-dependent VEGFR1 expression and constitutive VEGFR2 signaling in infantile hemangioma. Nat Med. 2008;14(11):1236–46.
96. Wu JK, Adepoju O, De Silva D, Baribault K, Boscolo E, Bischoff J, Kitajewski J. A switch in Notch gene expression parallels stem cell to endothelial transition in infantile hemangioma. Angiogenesis. 2010;13(1):15–23.
97. Boscolo E, Bischoff J. Vasculogenesis in infantile hemangioma. Angiogenesis. 2009;12(2): 197–207.
98. Boye E, Yu Y, Paranya G, Mulliken JB, Olsen BR, Bischoff J. Clonality and altered behavior of endothelial cells from hemangiomas. J Clin Invest. 2001;107(6):745–52.
99. Hoeger PH. Infantile haemangioma: new aspects on the pathogenesis of the most common skin tumour in children. Br J Dermatol. 2011;164(2):234–5.
100. Uihlein LC, Liang MG, Mulliken JB. Pathogenesis of infantile hemangiomas. Pediatr Ann. 2012;41(8):1–6.
101. North PE, Waner M, Mizeracki A, Mihm Jr MC. GLUT1: a newly discovered immunohistochemical marker for juvenile hemangiomas. Hum Pathol. 2000;31(1):11–22.
102. North PE, Waner M, Mizeracki A, Mrak RE, Nicholas R, Kincannon J, Suen JY, Mihm Jr MC. A unique microvascular phenotype shared by juvenile hemangiomas and human placenta. Arch Dermatol. 2001;137(5):559–70.
103. Barnes CM, Christison-Lagay EA, Folkman J. The placenta theory and the origin of infantile hemangioma. Lymphat Res Biol. 2007;5(4):245–55.
104. Barnes CM, Huang S, Kaipainen A, Sanoudou D, Chen EJ, Eichler GS, Guo Y, Yu Y, Ingber DE, Mulliken JB, Beggs AH, Folkman J, Fishman SJ. Evidence by molecular profiling for a placental origin of infantile hemangioma. Proc Natl Acad Sci U S A. 2005;102(52):19097–102.
105. Ritter MR, Butschek RA, Friedlander M, Friedlander SF. Pathogenesis of infantile haemangioma: new molecular and cellular insights. Expert Rev Mol Med. 2007;9(32):1–19.
106. Garzon MC, Drolet BA, Baselga E, Chamlin SL, Haggstrom AN, Horii K, Lucky AW, Mancini AJ, Metry DW, Newell B, Nopper AJ, Frieden IJ. Comparison of infantile hemangiomas in preterm and term infants: a prospective study. Arch Dermatol. 2008;144(9): 1231–2.
107. Haggstrom AN, Drolet BA, Baselga E, Chamlin SL, Garzon MC, Horii KA, Lucky AW, Mancini AJ, Metry DW, Newell B, Nopper AJ, Frieden IJ. Prospective study of infantile hemangiomas: demographic, prenatal, and perinatal characteristics. J Pediatr. 2007;150(3):291–4.
108. Burton BK, Schulz CJ, Angle B, Burd LI. An increased incidence of haemangiomas in infants born following chorionic villus sampling (CVS). Prenat Diagn. 1995;15(3):209–14.
109. Kaplan P, Normandin Jr J, Wilson GN, Plauchu H, Lippman A, Vekemans M. Malformations and minor anomalies in children whose mothers had prenatal diagnosis: comparison between CVS and amniocentesis. Am J Med Genet. 1990;37(3):366–70.
110. Pittman KM, Losken HW, Kleinman ME, Marcus JR, Blei F, Gurtner GC, Marchuk DA. No evidence for maternal-fetal microchimerism in infantile hemangioma: a molecular genetic investigation. J Invest Dermatol. 2006;126(11):2533–8.

111. Kleinman ME, Blei F, Gurtner GC. Circulating endothelial progenitor cells and vascular anomalies. Lymphat Res Biol. 2005;3(4):234–9.

112. Hamlat A, Adn M, Pasqualini E, Brassier G, Askar B. Pathophysiology of capillary haemangioma growth after birth. Med Hypotheses. 2005;64(6):1093–6.

113. Colonna V, Resta L, Napoli A, Bonifazi E. Placental hypoxia and neonatal haemangioma: clinical and histological observations. Br J Dermatol. 2010;162(1):208–9.

114. Lopez Gutierrez JC, Avila LF, Sosa G, Patron M. Placental anomalies in children with infantile hemangioma. Pediatr Dermatol. 2007;24(4):353–5.

115. Ahrens WA, Ridenour 3rd RV, Caron BL, Miller DV, Folpe AL. GLUT-1 expression in mesenchymal tumors: an immunohistochemical study of 247 soft tissue and bone neoplasms. Hum Pathol. 2008;39(10):1519–26.

116. Feldser D, Agani F, Iyer NV, Pak B, Ferreira G, Semenza GL. Reciprocal positive regulation of hypoxia-inducible factor 1alpha and insulin-like growth factor 2. Cancer Res. 1999;59(16):3915–8.

117. Herbert A, Ng H, Jessup W, Kockx M, Cartland S, Thomas SR, Hogg PJ, Wargon O. Hypoxia regulates the production and activity of glucose transporter-1 and indoleamine 2,3-dioxygenase in monocyte-derived endothelial-like cells: possible relevance to infantile haemangioma pathogenesis. Br J Dermatol. 2011;164(2):308–15.

118. Ritter MR, Reinisch J, Friedlander SF, Friedlander M. Myeloid cells in infantile hemangioma. Am J Pathol. 2006;168(2):621–8.

119. Bischoff J. Monoclonal expansion of endothelial cells in hemangioma: an intrinsic defect with extrinsic consequences? Trends Cardiovasc Med. 2002;12(5):220–4.

120. Allen RC, Zoghbi HY, Moseley AB, Rosenblatt HM, Belmont JW. Methylation of HpaII and HhaI sites near the polymorphic CAG repeat in the human androgen-receptor gene correlates with X chromosome inactivation. Am J Hum Genet. 1992;51(6):1229–39.

121. Walter JW, North PE, Waner M, Mizeracki A, Blei F, Walker JW, Reinisch JF, Marchuk DA. Somatic mutation of vascular endothelial growth factor receptors in juvenile hemangioma. Genes Chromosomes Cancer. 2002;33(3):295–303.

122. Dadras SS, North PE, Bertoncini J, Mihm MC, Detmar M. Infantile hemangiomas are arrested in an early developmental vascular differentiation state. Mod Pathol. 2004;17(9):1068–79.

123. Friedlander SF, Ritter MR, Friedlander M. Recent progress in our understanding of the pathogenesis of infantile hemangiomas. Lymphat Res Biol. 2005;3(4):219–25.

124. Ritter MR, Moreno SK, Dorrell MI, Rubens J, Ney J, Friedlander DF, Bergman J, Cunningham BB, Eichenfield L, Reinisch J, Cohen S, Veccione T, Holmes R, Friedlander SF, Friedlander M. Identifying potential regulators of infantile hemangioma progression through large-scale expression analysis: a possible role for the immune system and indoleamine 2,3 dioxygenase (IDO) during involution. Lymphat Res Biol. 2003;1(4):291–9.

125. Azzopardi S, Wright TC. Novel strategies for managing infantile hemangiomas: a review. Ann Plast Surg. 2012;68(2):226–8.

126. Mabeta P, Pepper MS. Hemangiomas – current therapeutic strategies. Int J Dev Biol. 2011;55(4–5):431–7.

127. Ezekowitz RA, Mulliken JB, Folkman J. Interferon alfa-2a therapy for life-threatening hemangiomas of infancy. N Engl J Med. 1992;326(22):1456–63.

128. Barlow CF, Priebe CJ, Mulliken JB, Barnes PD, Mac Donald D, Folkman J, Ezekowitz RA. Spastic diplegia as a complication of interferon Alfa-2a treatment of hemangiomas of infancy. J Pediatr. 1998;132(3 Pt 1):527–30.

129. Luo QF, Zhao FY. The effects of Bleomycin A5 on infantile maxillofacial haemangioma. Head Face Med. 2011;7:11.

130. Leaute-Labreze C, Dumas de la Roque E, Hubiche T, Boralevi F, Thambo JB, Taieb A. Propranolol for severe hemangiomas of infancy. N Engl J Med. 2008;358(24):2649–51.

131. Menezes MD, McCarter R, Greene EA, Bauman NM. Status of propranolol for treatment of infantile hemangioma and description of a randomized clinical trial. Ann Otol Rhinol Laryngol. 2011;120(10):686–95.

132. Storch CH, Hoeger PH. Propranolol for infantile haemangiomas: insights into the molecular mechanisms of action. Br J Dermatol. 2010;163(2):269–74.
133. Greenberger S, Boscolo E, Adini I, Mulliken JB, Bischoff J. Corticosteroid suppression of VEGF-A in infantile hemangioma-derived stem cells. N Engl J Med. 2010;362(11):1005–13.
134. Edgerton MT. The treatment of hemangiomas: with special reference to the role of steroid therapy. Ann Surg. 1976;183(5):517–32.
135. Batta K, Goodyear HM, Moss C, Williams HC, Hiller L, Waters R. Randomised controlled study of early pulsed dye laser treatment of uncomplicated childhood haemangiomas: results of a 1-year analysis. Lancet. 2002;360(9332):521–7.
136. Admani S, Krakowski AC, Nelson JS, Eichenfield LF, Friedlander SF. Beneficial effects of early pulsed dye laser therapy in individuals with infantile hemangiomas. Dermatol Surg. 2012;38(10):1732–8.

Index

© Springer-Verlag London Ltd. 2017   173
J.L. Arbiser (ed.), *Angiogenesis-Based Dermatology*,
DOI 10.1007/978-1-4471-7314-4